BABA MAGAZINE

The magazine for men who care about their health.

I0500439

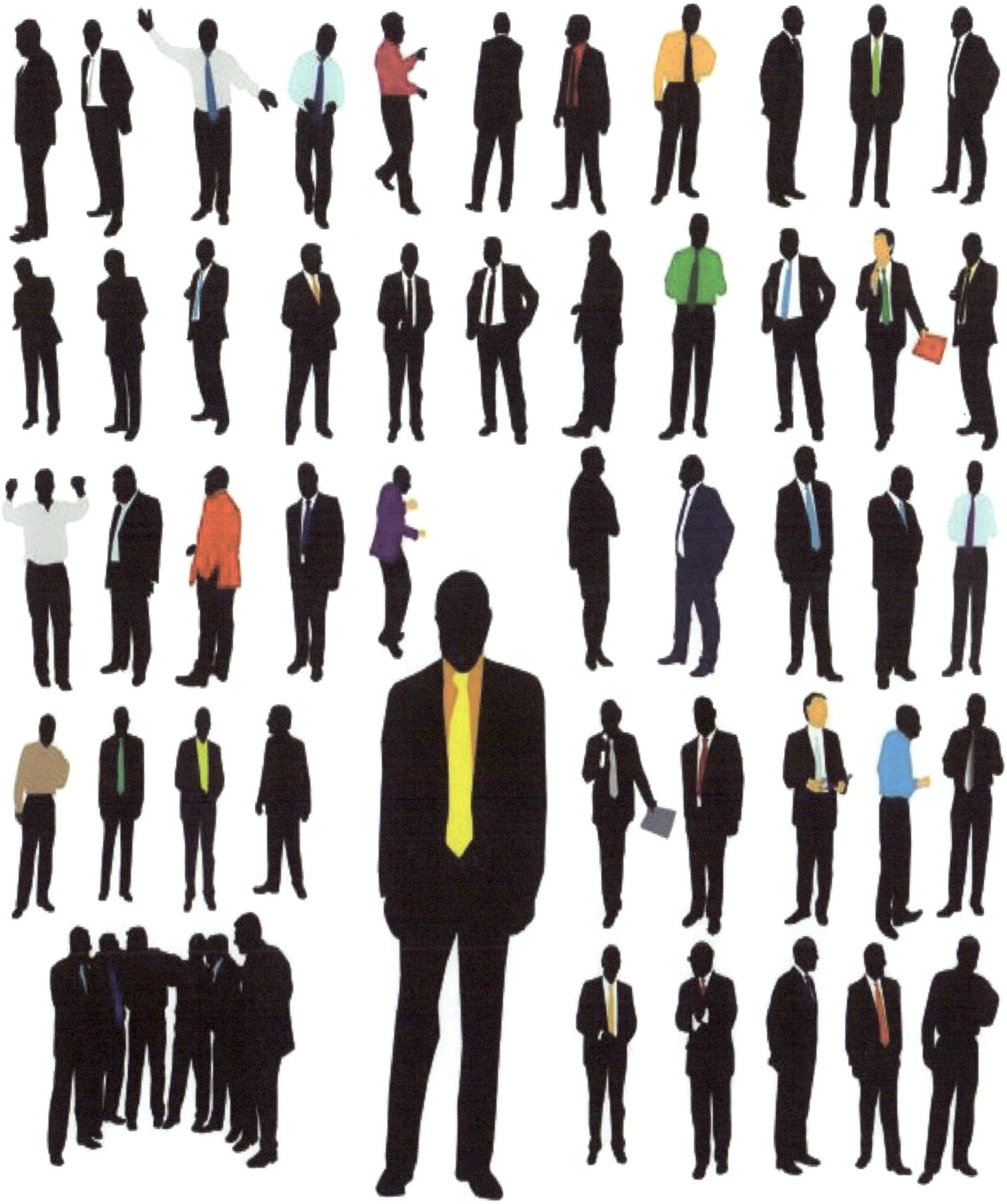

Baba Magazine

9205 Rue Bayne, Lasalle. Montreal H8R 2H1 QC CA Email: babamagazine@gmail.com

To advertise in the magazine, contact the Editor.

Subscription $120 annually.

Available in print and e-zine

Printed by Amazon Kindle Direct Printers

In this Issue:

Editorial

Welcome BABA, dad, father! This is your magazine! The magazine that contains information that will help you look after your health and the health of younger men in your life. Don't miss an issue and do not wait to be told half-truths by other men at the club. Get your own copy of this magazine and read about your health, promoting good health, restoring health after periods of overlooking growing problems and maintaining good health.

This magazine will help you select the right health choices in life and gives you an opportunity to ask questions about your health So, go on, grab the opportunity and ask about those aspects of health that worry you most, that give you sleepless nights, the issues you wouldn't talk about to a friend. BABA will respond to all your questions with well researched up to date professional health information, not pub tales!

BABA is aware of other important things in life men value and BABA will bring these into the magazine for your enjoyment. If you have a subject you want addressed, just write to BABA requesting topics you want included in the magazine. Enjoy the magazine! Enjoy good health!

Editor

Nester Kadzviti Murira

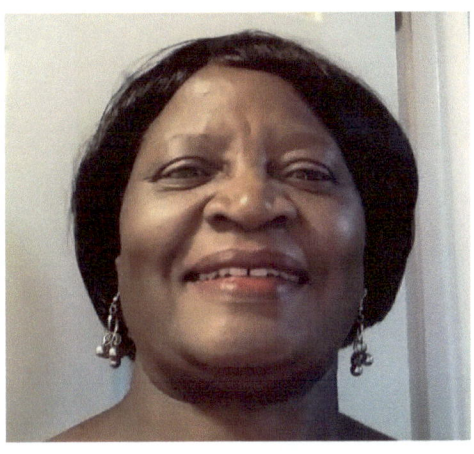

BOYS TO MEN

Growing up is a process of life that starts at birth and consists of several phases. Growing up can be likened to a journey with significant landmarks and signposts. The most important of these landmarks is called Puberty. After this a young man proceeds to the signposts of an adolescent then a young man who subsequently progresses to become an adult man.

Ideally this process or journey with its signposts should be a guided process in which adult men induct younger men step by step into adulthood through informed discussion and mentoring as well as through examples that the young man observes and emulates in life. This involves a lot of learning through observation.

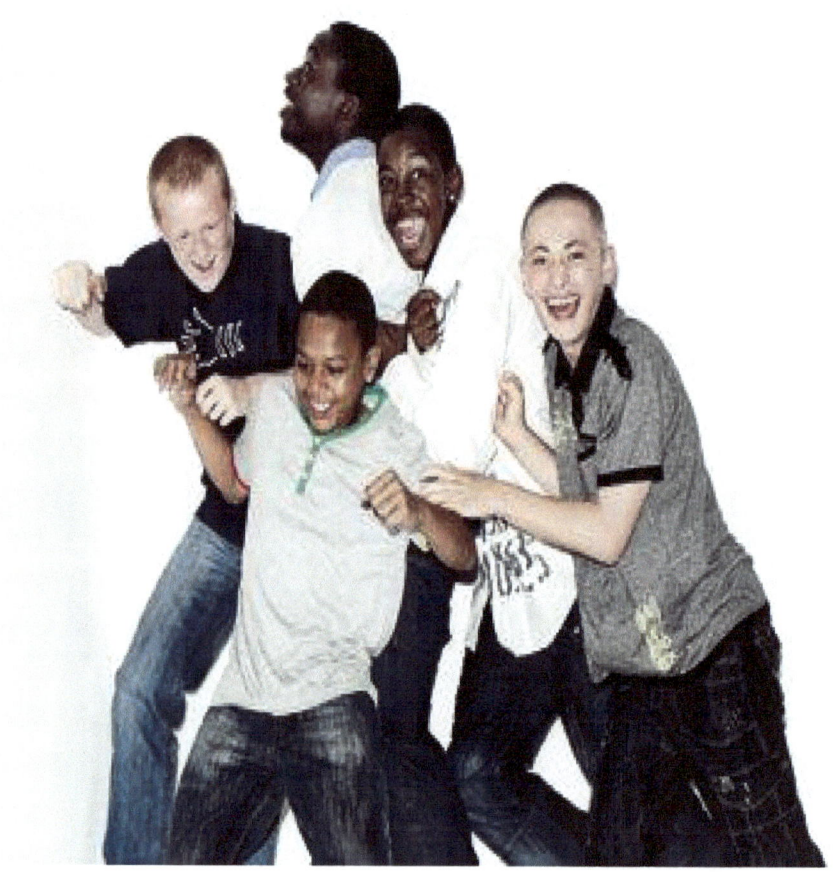

LANDMARK PUBERTY

Puberty is the stage of transition from childhood to an adolescent. It is brought about by two in the boychild's body namely:

- Growth Hormone or Somatotrophic Hormone and

- Sex Hormones or Gonadotrophic Hormones.

Both these hormones are produced by a small but very powerful organ commonly referred to as the brain's master gland or the pituitary gland in medical terms. This small organ sits at the base of the skull below the brain.

The Growth hormone is in the child's body from birth but increases in amounts at puberty while the sex hormones are produced in increasing amounts from the age of eight years.

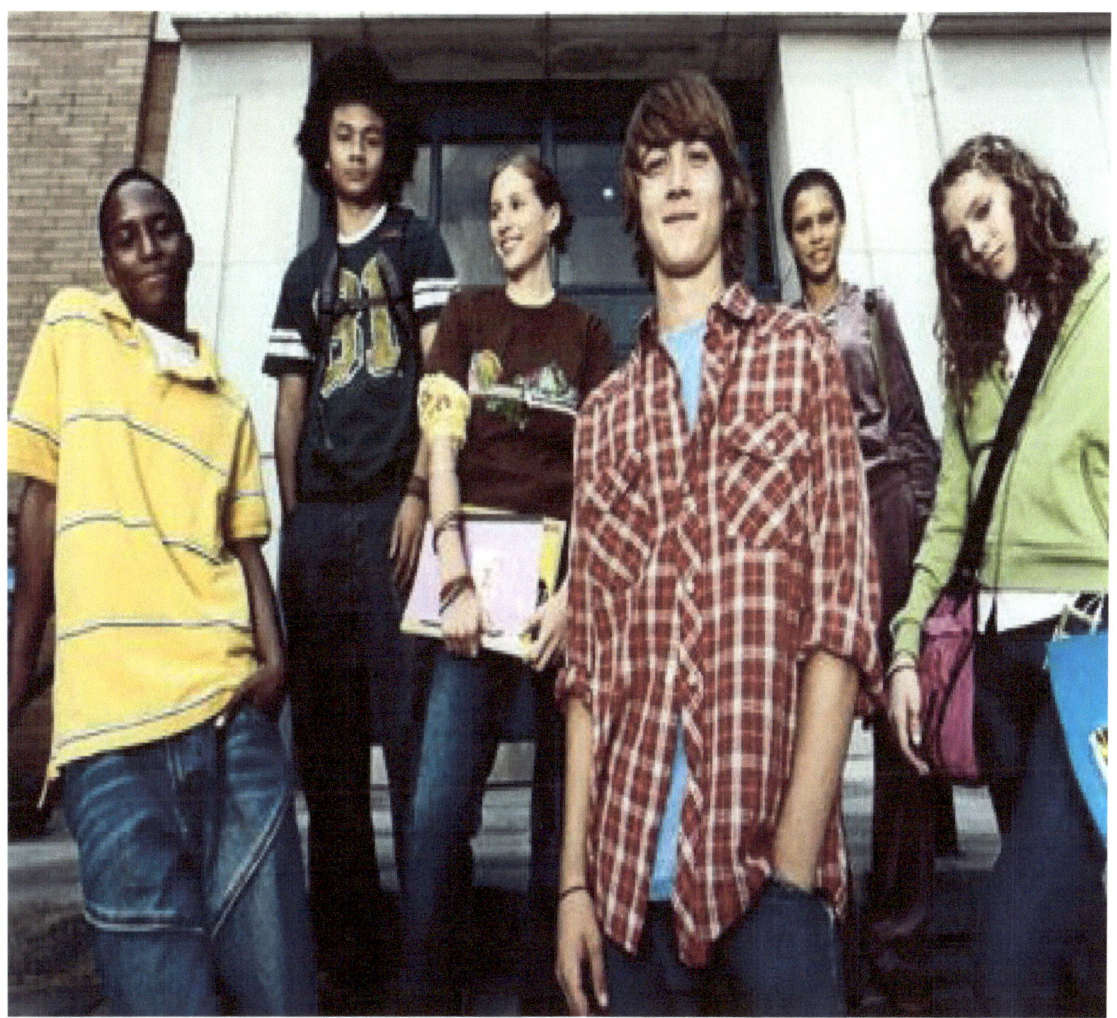

Physical Changes in Boys

The two hormones bring a package of changes to the young boy's body designed to influence the male body's development.
The Growth Hormone takes care of growth.

- There is a rapid physical growth that changes or transforms a young boy into an adolescent then into a young man. The changes are observable and influence the growth of long bones and development of a broad chest and shoulders.

This growth spurt may bring about a mixture of confusion and excitement in a young person who becomes aware of the physical changes in his body.

- The growth changes are in all parts of the body and in all the systems of the body.

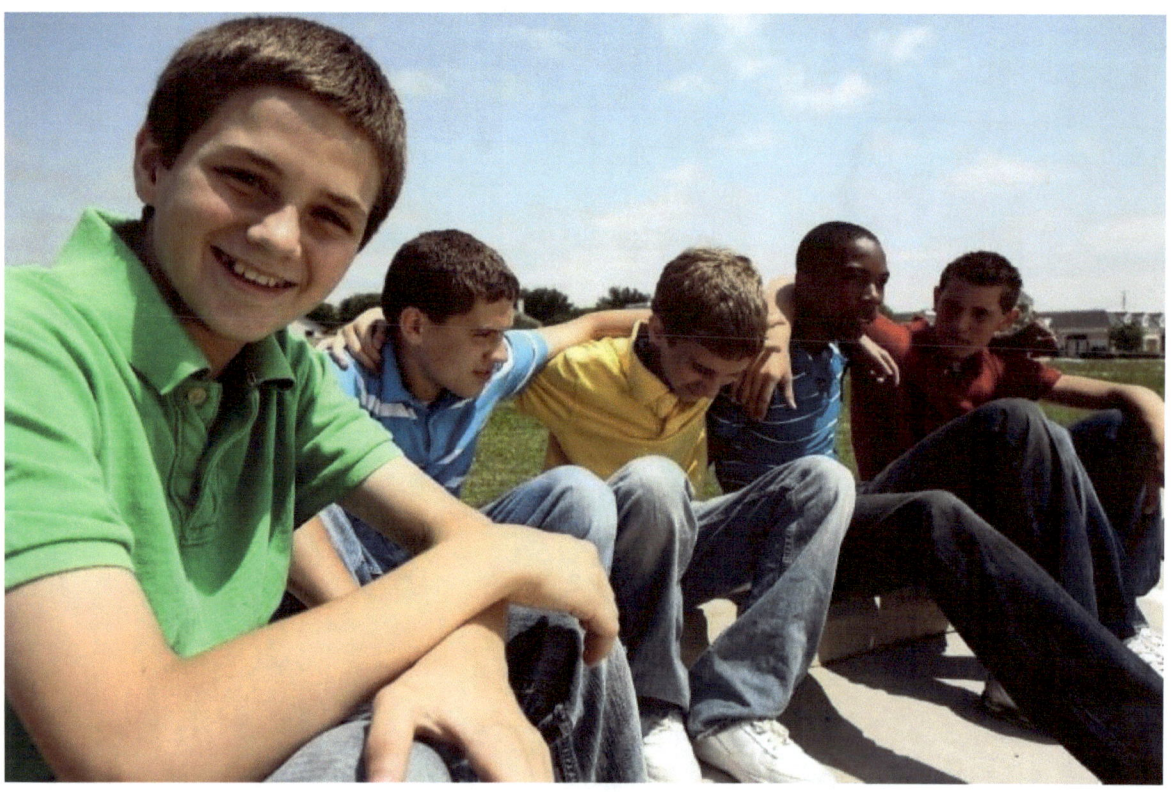

This is the opportune time for the parent to explain what all the changes mean and how to manage the changes responsibly. From the time the changes begin to show, the lessons of adulthood must go on and intensify as the adolescent continues to grow.

The Gonadotrophins or Sex Hormones

- These hormones directly influence the male reproductive system to become fully developed.

The testes mature and enlarge and descend from the abdomen through a small opening in the groin, **the inguinal canal** to sit in the scrotum, a pouch or sac below the groins where they should remain for the rest of the male adult life. Sometimes testes remain in the abdomen, an abnormal situation called *undescended testes.* This is corrected through surgery. If the condition is not corrected early, the young man may have infertility.

It is important that at puberty young men feel the little balls or testes in the scrotum. It is advised that an adolescent reports to health personnel if the scrotal sac remains empty when all the other signs of puberty are present.

- In the scrotal pouch or sac, the testes are kept at a temperature that is below the body temperature to enable them to function normally.

- The testes produce spermatozoa or the male seed. It is advisable that young men avoid tight underwear that generates heat and alter scrotal temperature and, should opt for loose airy underwear. Excessive heat to the scrotum, the sac containing the men's balls, slows sperm production.

**Young men who work in furnaces and long-distance drivers of haulages trucks should take time to cool their body temperatures.
There are two sex hormones necessary in a man's body.

The Follicle Stimulating hormone (FSH), one of the sex hormones from the brain, stimulates the testes to become active and fully functional glands that produce the male seed, *the spermatozoa.*

Spermatozoa swim in a white fluid, *semen*, which is produced in the testes in limited amounts and most of the semen is produced by one large gland, the prostate gland, which surrounds the urethra.

The Interstitial Cell Stimulating hormone, (ICSH) is the second male sex hormone which **stimulates the testes or (the balls), to produce the male sex hormone, TESTOSTERONE.**

TESTOSTERONE **is responsible for the maleness in a young man**, marked by growth of internal male sexual organs, male characteristics, and male sexual behaviors.

- Boys will begin to grow a little hair on the chin which will later become beard. Hair also grows in armpits and on the pubic area.

This is the time to talk about armpit and pubic hair cleanliness. Armpits catch sweat which dries producing a nasty body odor. Removing hairs in the armpit and use of anti-perspirant deodorants removes the odor and makes a young man acceptable by others and gives him confidence.

- Body odor does not disappear by just a shower, a deodorant is a 'must have' for every young person from puberty onwards.

Testosterone together with the Growth hormone influence

- The young man's voice deepens, a development commonly known as *'breaking of voice'* and the voice box or Adam's apple becomes visibly enlarged.

- Muscular development in the young man. The typical broad shoulders, the strong male muscles and the strong thigh muscles.

- There is an observable increase in height caused by lengthening of long bones.

Young men's appetite naturally increases at puberty to enable the young man to develop physically and in strength.

Testosterone **is responsible for sexual desire,**

- The need to attract and be noticed by the opposite sex and

- Testosterone triggers the urge to experiment with the developed organs, hence the need for adolescent sexual health education around puberty for both young men and women.

- The drive to physically engage in sexual activity. Boys dream of erotic scenes and discharge semen with spermatozoa in their sleep, commonly referred to as *wet dreams.*

Should a young man have sexual intercourse from this stage of development and onwards, he can become a father, a 'Teenage parent!'

- It is important that young men are guided to get the relevant social skills to present themselves in an acceptable manner to the opposite sex and avoid throwing themselves on young women.

- Guidance is needed to help the adolescent cope with the outpour of hormones in their bodies. The world is sick of stories of young men who cannot control their hormones and abuse little girls and boys at this stage.

Testosterone drive can be **redirected into chores that require energy** including working out in the gym, sprinting ball games and any game that saps energy. A cold shower is a remedy to cooling down nerves and wild ideas.

From Puberty onwards, parents have a young man at hand.

- It is important that parents talk to young men about restraint. Young men should not depend on instinct to express themselves neither should young men learn male behaviors from friends. Boys who learn through instinct and friends usually make a mess of their relationships.

- Guidance of young men into manhood by a mentor who could be his father or an older brother or a guardian cannot be over-emphasized. A young man must be groomed for the future stages beyond boyhood.

- Young men should be engaged in discussion of prevention of unwanted pregnancy!

- **The discussion must include the use of a condom.**

In some families, young men may become men without observing responsible and essential guidance on socially accepted attitudes, language, behaviors acceptable in society.

In most cultures, girls are groomed following well-defined expected behaviors and skills acquisition along the lifeline. Girls are given dolls to care for, little pots to learn to cook, brooms and dusters to learn to clean the house and surroundings, chores that the mother instills in the young girl from an early stage in life to prepare her for motherhood.

Just like the female species train a girlchild to be a woman by exposing her and enabling her to practice feminine roles, men should do the same.

Young women sometimes are shocked to find what they have at hand is not what they expected and desired. It is important that mature men take the responsibility of mentoring young men from the transitional period of puberty to manhood.

Fathers must have a good relationship with their sons so that they can discuss manly topics freely along the lifeline, facts of life and expected, acceptable behaviors in adulthood.

It is best that a child learns facts of life from a parent, a close relative or guided lessons in churches, youth clubs and colleges than from friends.

A family, and a parent should be responsible for branding their child.

Parents must answer the young men's questions honestly and not evade questions or leave the adolescent to learn through trial and error or discovery. A parent who handles the questions himself ensures that his child gets correct information. Don't allow your child to get information from friends. Your child may be fed half- truths and lies.

Beliefs and Myths

There are untrue and uninformed beliefs and myths that circulate in societies that may mislead young people in trying to understand sexuality. It is important that young people seek answers to the questions and anxieties they may have from informed sources.

Forward your questions to BABA magazine and every question will be addressed.

MEN AND SEXUAL STABILITY

There are some cultures which insist that young men marry a virgin. This is commendable but young people must be assisted to control their behaviors and manage the feelings brought about by the influx of hormones at puberty.

Young men must be groomed to stick to one partner right from the outset instead of running everywhere and acquiring reputations of leaving no dress unturned before they get married. This is a typical example of loss of control, lack of proper guidance and lack of respect for the opposite sex. It is not being macho.

Mature men too must show control and be exemplary so that young people have decent role models. It is disgraceful for elderly men to go back to the cradles to pick the ages of their daughters for sexual partners! The rapist is doing his rounds too! So where do virgins come from? The buck stops with you guys! Virginity is important in both partners. Young men must be virgins if they desire a virgin marry. Two virgins on the wedding night is a fair deal!

Virginity at marriage increases trust between partners and reduces the incidence of sexually transmitted diseases including HIV and AIDS in married couples. Staying a virgin till the wedding day is about self-control, self-respect and respect for your partner. It is not cool to bed many women. That type of behavior says a lot about the individual. It means the guy does not know what he is looking for. The guy has an unstable character and cannot be trusted. He cheats. He certainly would not rank very high as a marriage partner.

When can such a person be expected to stop that behavior and focus on giving all his attention to one woman, his wife? What exactly are men looking for when they want to bed several women? Could it be that some men mistake love for lust? If it is love, such men are after, surely, they can get it in abundance from one sexual partner. Women get better and mellow with age like wine. If a man has several girlfriends before marriage, and fathers several children out of wedlock, is that man capable of loving one woman after marriage? Can he become a faithful husband to one woman, his wife? Surely his attention will always be divided, and it is possible he will continue to cheat on his partner throughout his life.

Young men are driven into marriage by a desire to have a sexual partner in their beds 365 days of the year. But, the same young men fall short of deep enduring love as expected by women. It is the responsibility of mature men and fathers to advise young men to respect their bodies and be faithful loving partners to their spouses. Mature men should prepare young men for manly responsibilities.

Mature men too, have a responsibility to be exemplary to young men. It is not dignified of mature men to be jostling with young men on the hunting field for young women to bed. Can any man claim to have anything to show after the years of *quickies* in odd places with young women?

Let's talk about it.

Sexual Responsibility

Responsible sexual behavior is enhanced by knowledge about one's sexual organs and how they function. Sexual responsibility is about understanding the consequences of sexual activity. It includes taking precautions to prevent negative consequences of sexual activity such as unwanted unplanned pregnancies and contracting sexually transmitted diseases. It takes a real man to accept the responsibilities that come with sexual activity. Some young men just want to jump into bed with a woman then walk away without a second thought about it. What if she falls pregnant or has sexually transmitted diseases? What if she contracts the disease the man has? Thinking about these questions, communicating about precautions before the action and taking the precautions is sexual responsibility.

Why do some men refuse to accept a pregnancy they are fully aware that they were responsible for? Please do the world a favor and only engage in sexual activity after considering and accepting the responsibilities. Participate in prevention of pregnancy if you don't want responsibility.

Sexual Precautions

There are several methods of contraception available for both men and women to prevent unwanted pregnancy or delay pregnancy. There are methods of contraception that also prevent sexually transmitted diseases like the male and female condom.

If a man feels that he is ready for sexual activity, then he must be man enough to take precautions to prevent unwanted unpleasant and serious consequences of irresponsible sexual behaviour.

It is important that one gets himself one partner and sticks to his partner. It is easier then to plan and discuss with partner on suitable methods to delay pregnancy and together the couple can seek reliable information about these methods from health personnel.

There is no reason why one's partner should fall pregnant if she does not want to or if you as the partner do not want her to. It is equally a man's responsibility to prevent pregnancy as much as it is a woman's.

The Condom

THE CONDOM is the only contraceptive method for both men and women that prevents both sexually transmitted infections including HIV and unwanted, unplanned, pregnancy.

- The condom is the best method for young people who do not wish to start taking hormones early in life.

- The condom does not need a prescription or measurement of one's body structures. One size fits them all whether you are well endowed, or you are small.

- **The condom is readily available** in shops, chemists, the doctor's rooms, and health centres. The condom is the best method when a couple wishes to prevent or delay pregnancy. There are readily available from most shops at the asking.

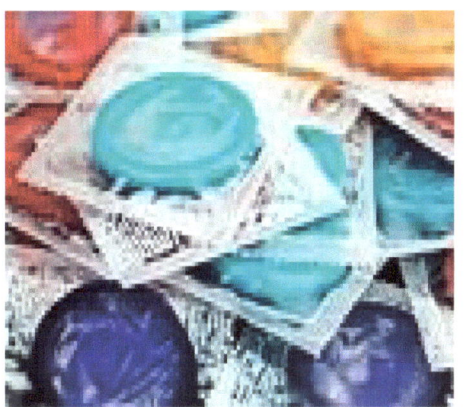

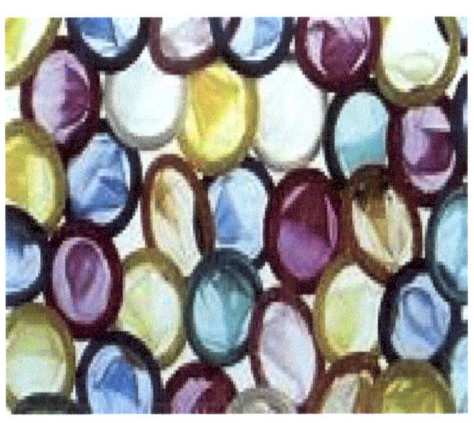

- The condom is easily the best method to use while one's partner recovers from a pregnancy as one does not need to see health personnel to start using it.

- The condom can also be used when your partner is starting on a hormone method for the first two weeks to allow the hormone blood levels to reach safe levels that prevent pregnancy.

- The condom is *the only method that prevents pregnancy as well as protecting an individual from contracting sexually transmitted diseases.*

How does one use the male condom?

- The man must wear the condom when aroused and before the sexual act.

- Your partner can help to apply it as part of foreplay.

- There is no need to apply oil or jel on the man, the condom is well lubricated.

- It is important to hold the top of the condom as one ease out of his partner to prevent spillage of semen onto the partner's organs.

- Wrap the condom in tissue paper and flush it in the toilet or dispose of it in the rubbish bin.

- Use a condom once for one act and dispose of it.

- Do not wash or use repeatedly.

- Unused condoms must be stored away from heat and the sun. Rubber is weakened and destroyed by heat.

- There is no reason why a man and his partner should contract sexually transmitted diseases because **the condom is available everywhere.**

Female condom

There is a condom for your partner as well.

- The female condom prevents both pregnancy and sexually transmitted infections.

- The female condom must be worn before the sexual act just like the male condom.

There are other methods like the **Foams** and **Pessaries** that a young woman can introduce inside her female organ before sexual intercourse. The foam and pessary must be repeated should the couple feel they need to have another sexual act.

Women have many other alternative reliable choices of methods of contraception that they can use but there is no reason why a man cannot share the responsibility and fully participate in prevention of sexually transmitted infections and unwanted pregnancy.

It is important to check with one's partner that she is protected from an unwanted pregnancy before a sexual act.

If both partners take the necessary precautions, then sexually transmitted diseases and unwanted pregnancy can be avoided.

SEXUAL ABUSE

Sexual abuse includes touching, fondling, patting, of an individual's body, contact with another person's sexual organs either by touching or penetration or forcing oneself on an individual or illicit sexual assault without consent.

- Anyone including trusted members of families, members of society entrusted with the care of children in schools, and refugee camps as well as social deviants and perverts have been reported to sexually abuse young people.
- There is no need for men to behave in such irresponsible sexual behavior.
- Real men, ask mature women for a sexual relationship.
- Real men control their sexual desires and do not take advantage of innocent helpless children or young girls.
- Sex is for adults who both know the consequences of their behavior and who enjoy the sexual act. Children are not sexual, they don't understand why an adult hurts them. Some children are exposed to infections like gonorrhea, sore throat through oral sex, syphilis and syphilitic body rashes that maybe mistaken for eczema and the dreaded HIV infection.

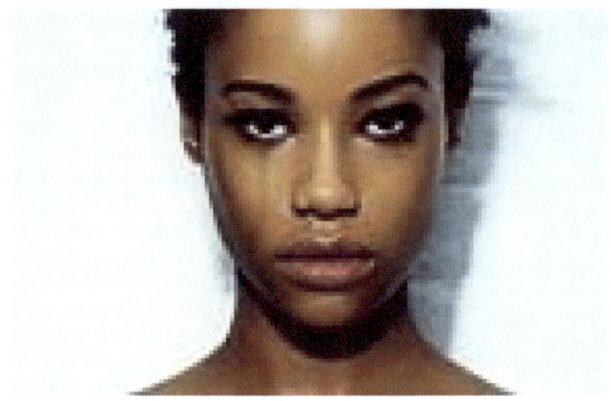

- Sexually abusing children confuses children, changes their characters, makes them timid individuals and takes away their innocence.

- Responsible men control their sexual desire until they find a woman that they agree with to have a sexual act. Sexual act is between adults. Do not hurt innocent little children by forcing yourself onto them! It is cruel, inhuman behavior that is punishable by law. Sexual activity with a child below the age of eighteen is taking advantage of the young person.

- Sexually abusing children is punishable by law.

- If you know anyone abusing childrenplease report the culprit to Police.

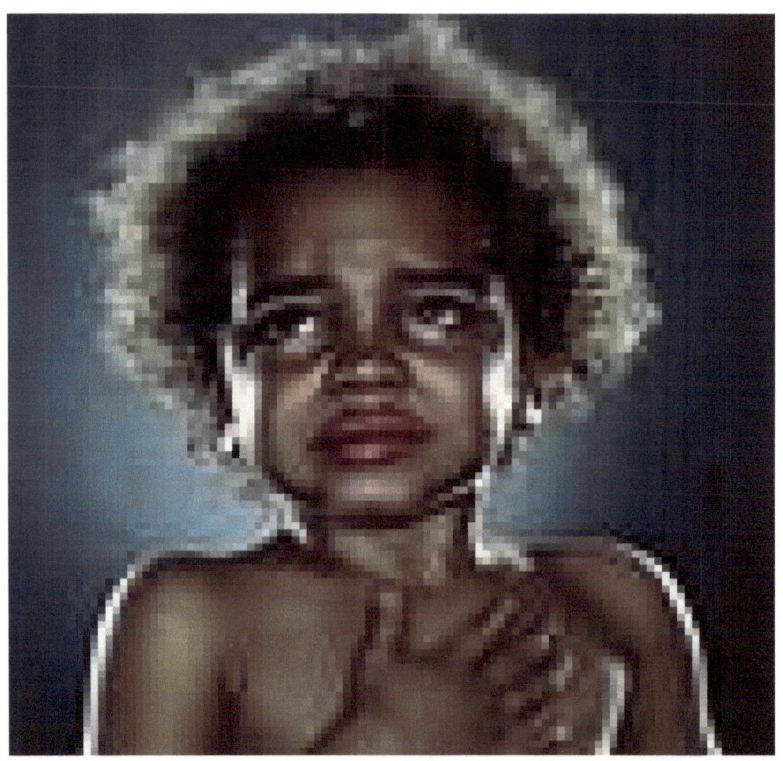

INCEST

Incestuous relationships are sexual relationship between related people or close family members.

- Parents, guardians, brothers and uncles entrusted with the welfare of a girl child **should never** take advantage of the girl child! There are more women than men in the world! There are plenty of mature women looking for men and ready for a sexual act! Any man who wants a mature sexual partner can get one!

- Respect a relative. Don't behave like an animal which knows no boundaries. Don't force yourself on a relative; it makes you a pervert, undesirable in society and a sex offender.

- Some misguided family members believe incestuous relationships bring luck in business, in misfortune, and in illness. Sexual abuse of a relative does not bring any luck or relieve any illness; neither does it solve anyone's problems.

- Sexual abuse robs a young person of her innocence; it confuses the young person and may cause emotional instability.

- The young girl can be exposed to sexually transmitted diseases including the deadly HIV/AIDS. Don't hurt a child! Sexual intercourse is for adults not babies and children! Let children be children.

RAPE...

- Rape is forced sexual act without the consent of one partner. It is an offence and punishable by law.

- A woman should be able to freely choose her sexual partner.

- Sexual activity is more enjoyable if there is consent between mature people. Respect women! Women are not sex objects that men can use forcibly to relieve their desires! Women have a right to have sexual intercourse with a man of their choice.

- Decent enjoyable sexual intercourse is every person's right and that right must not be taken away from unsuspecting women by some misguided man who lacks control of his body!

- Rape does not make a man macho or desirable or respected. It makes a man an undesirable social deviant, a social outcast, a criminal.

- Women want to be respected and to have their rights of freedom of a sexual partner respected. It is possible for a man to control his desire for sex until he finds a mature person who is willing to engage in a sexual activity.

- If a man makes himself presentable, attractive, pleasant, he makes himself irresistible and can attract an equally attractive partner.

- There are perverts the world over who abduct young girls and take them in secluded places for the perverts' sexual needs.

- Take interest in who your daughter communicates with on internet, who she socializes with and what the subject of the communication is. Young girls can be lured by sexual perverts pretending to be their age mates and abducted through internet communication.

- It is important to know your daughter's friends and their parents. It cannot be overstated that young girls need close parental protection.

- It is safest to take your young girl to school and leave her in the school yard and make it your responsibility to collect her from school.

- When you go shopping or for an outing with your daughter, keep your daughter within sight. When you are going away, ensure that you leave your daughter with people you know and trust

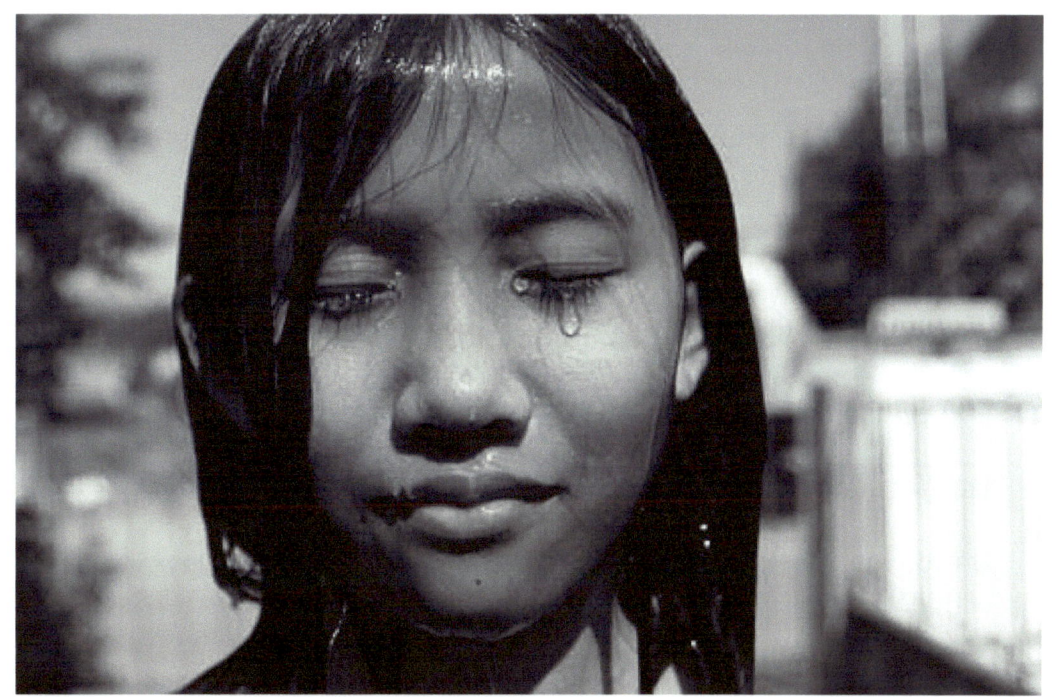

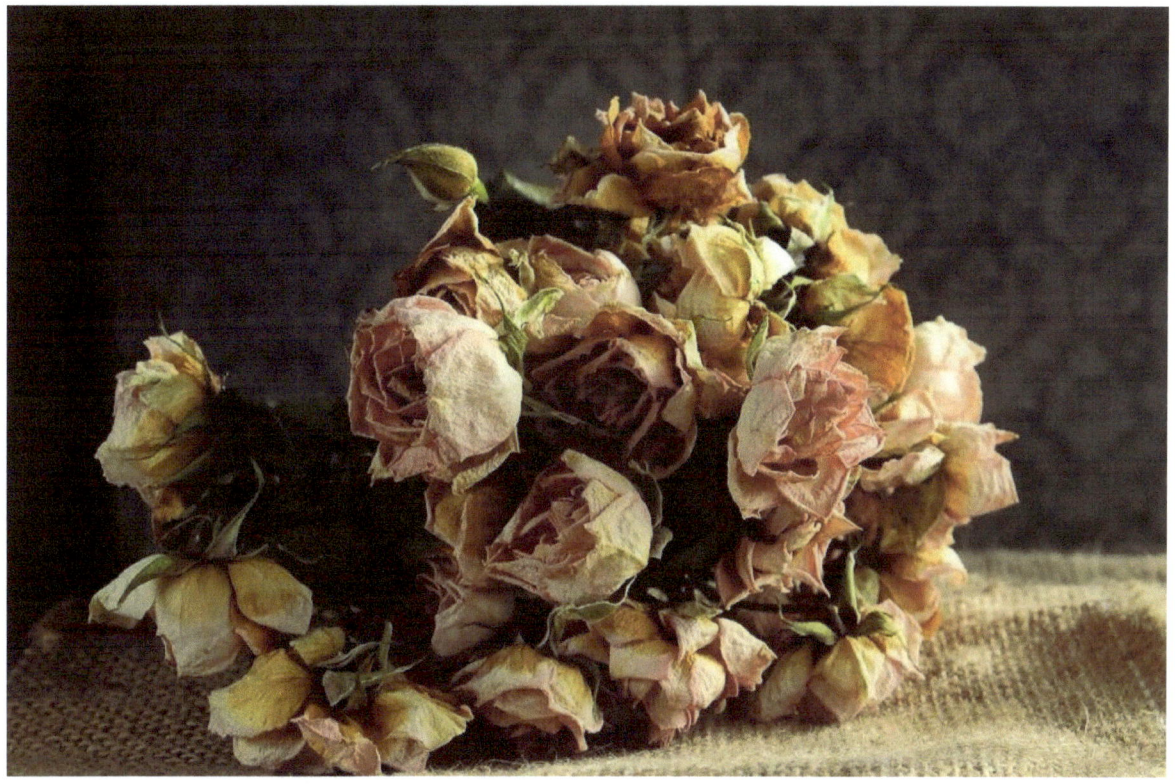

LET'S TALK BODY STRUCTURE

There is a growing problem among some men!

Your health is your responsibility! Today take a few minutes to look at yourself and make an honest self-assessment of yourself from head to toes.

Do you like the way you look in the mirror or on pictures?

Look at each part of your body objectively.

Do you look like you have a second chin? How does your neck look like? Can you turn with ease? Do your cheeks look like you have stuffed them with food?

Are you happy with your body so far?

Move down to your chest and assess your breathing. Do you wheeze and get breathless when walking?

How wide is your chest? Can your partner easily put her hands around you?
Are you always short of breath?

How wide is your upper arm? Do you see flab hanging from your forearms? Lift your arms as high as you can. How do your upper arms look like? Can you keep them straight up for a couple of minutes?

Is your belly falling onto your thighs?

Can you see your pubic hair? Do you need to lift flabs of your belly up as you wash? If you can't see your pubic hair while you are standing, your belly is out of control!

Is your belly threatening to pop out of your shirt? Have you bought clothes one size larger than before of late?

Do you struggle to button your shirt around the abdomen? **Must you breathe in to button the shirt?** Are your clothes getting tighter? If you have changed clothes sizes from large to x-large or to xx-large, and if you need a special tailor to make you special fits, you could be on the helm of the pot belly club! **You have added unwanted width on your belly!**

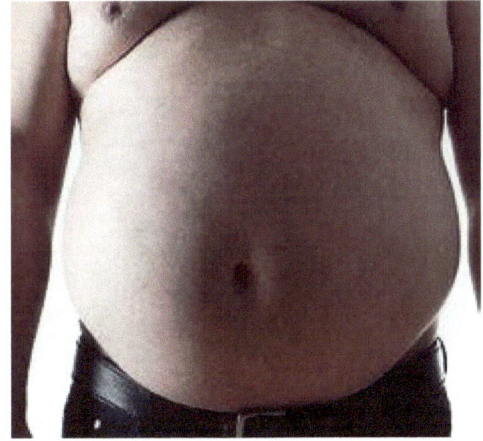

Can you see your belly through your buttoned shirt, do your shirt buttonholes look stretched and are the buttons threatening to fall off? You could be nursing a potbelly! If the threads of your favorite sweater are stretched over your belly, you have grown too big around the tummy.

Look at your body profile as you stand sideways in front of a mirror, if you look like a pregnant woman, you surely are inviting a health problem that is if you don't have a problem yet!

- Can you easily fit into your old jeans you bought last year?
- When shopping, do you look for the largest size of clothes on the rail?
- Do you shop in special shops for people like you?
- Do you find it difficult to bend over because the belly is in the way?
- Do you need a double seat?
- Can you walk briskly for fifty yards? Are you huffing and puffing like an old steam engine when you walk?
- Do you feel breathless after doing a small chore?
- Do you feel aches and pains in your joints? Do your shoes fit well?
- Do you need a motorized chair to do your shopping at the local grocery shop?
- Are you tipping your bathroom scales?
- Is your sex life dying or dead or do you leave your spouse to do all the work?
- If your answer is yes to some or all the above questions you need to get out of your recliner chair and join the gym for a healthy life! Lose that extra baggage; you don't need it!

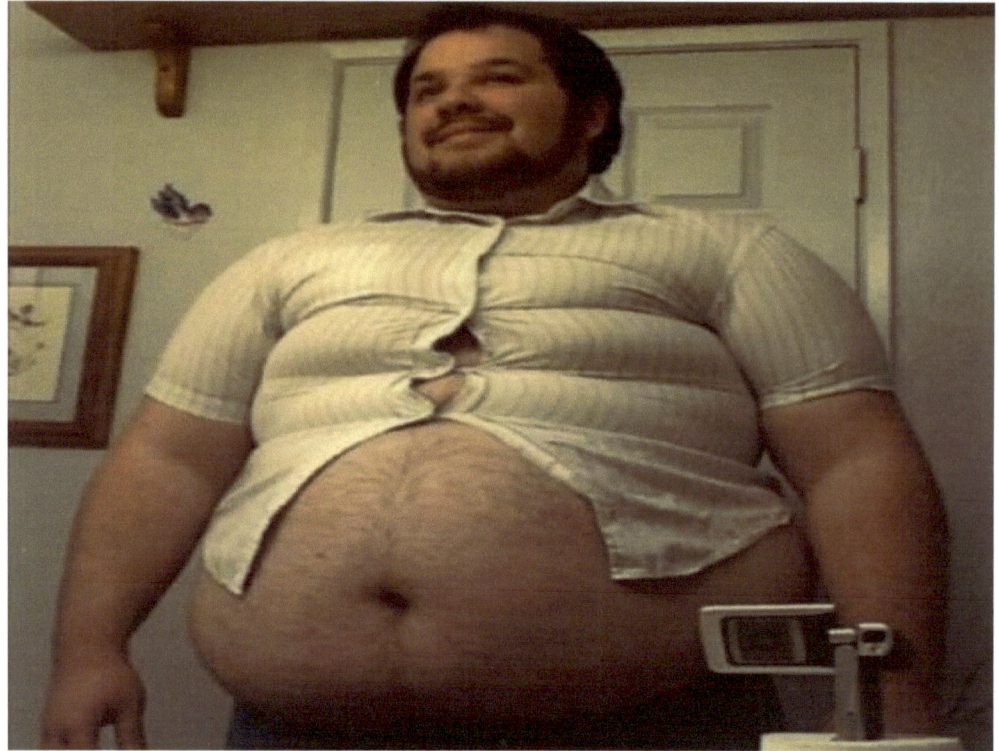

- **What causes a potbelly?**
- Men acquire their bellies from bad, uncontrolled eating.
- You don't have to eat everything on your plate. You can leave some food to eat the next day! If you want a lot of food, then fill your plate with more greens.
- Excessive alcohol consumption **is dangerous.** Beer contains loads of sugars. The more beer you take the more you are piling sugars into your body. These are converted to fat and stored under the skin especially around the belly and bums.
- Lack of exercise!

Eating and sleeping or eating and sitting to play video games, watch television all day into the small hours of the morning all promote obesity.

Unlike the general myth that big is a sign of affluence and good living, weight gain should be a real cause for concern. Excessive weight around your tummy is a load of health problems!

- A huge man with a potbelly looks untidy. Clothes don't fit well!
- A man with a big belly doesn't look attractive at all as he pushes around a big belly! Men like slim girls; the feeling is mutual! Women too like their men nice and shapely!

Why is excessive weight bad for you?

Big or overweight is not good living or comfort. It is good living gone bad!

An overweight man is likely to suffer from painful joints especially of the lower legs because the poor legs are carrying a heavy load and because the joints are suffering, they become swollen and painful.

Excessive weight strains your heart and you are in danger of a heart attack.

 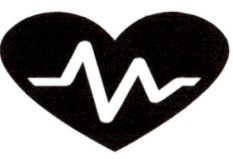

Excessive weight raises your Blood Pressure and high blood pressure may bring about a stroke.

You become a good candidate for breathing problems like Asthma.

Do you want to add a few more years to your life?

Do you love life? Excessive weight is giving up on life!

Excessive weight exposes you to Diabetes!.

When the body has extra starches that it does not need, the hormone that controls use and absorption of carbohydrate (insulin), becomes overwhelmed.

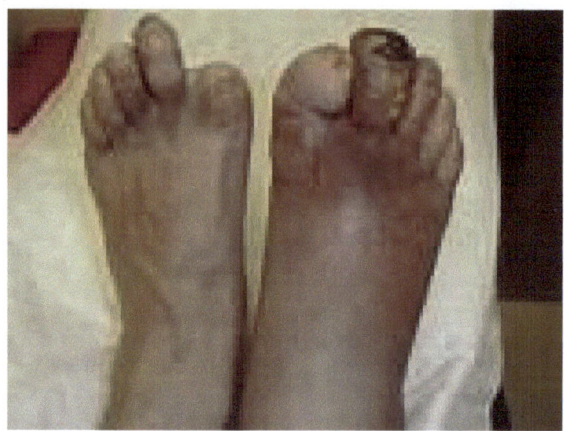

- A potbelly means there are heaps and heaps of fat around the stomach, the bowels, all the internal organs including around the heart and fat inside blood vessels!
- Fat does not stretch so the heart feels crowded and slowly gets tired.
- Blood does not flow well inside the fat padded blood vessels; the heart is taxed trying to push blood to the brain up the body and down to the toes against fat-lined blood vessels. **The result is High Blood Pressure!**

The above nasty uncomfortable health problems can be avoided by observing healthy habits.

A man needs to be active around the home and must be able to carry his weight easily when doing jobs around the home. You should be able to get up the ladder to fix the gutter, the leaking roof.

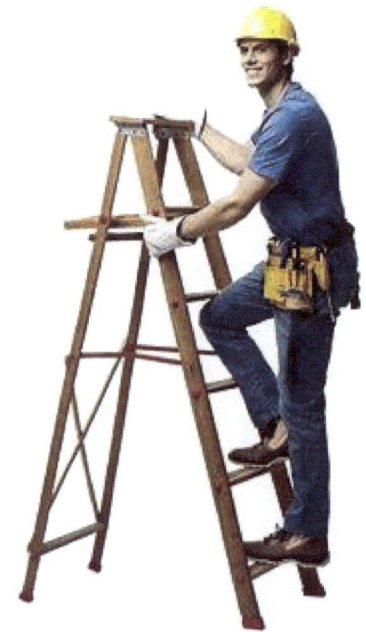

A healthy man must be able to play games with children or grandchildren.

Most important of all, a man must be able to perform his manly duties without risking a heart attack! Women don't like sloppy breathless men around them!

Make up your mind today and **shed off the unnecessary weight** you are carrying.

It is time to ACT now! **Get rid of the potbelly!**

Overweight is living dangerously! How can one lose the growing problem?

Lose that extra weight and start today! Help yourself control your weight:

- Avoid fatty roast meats,

- Cut down on white starchy foods like potatoes, rice, spaghetti, fufu, sadza

- Choose fruit instead of sweet dishes and desserts,

- Replace white bread with seeded or whole wheat bread

- **Eat sensibly!** Take small portions of food on your plate! If the food is already served on a plate, ask for a plate to offload what you don't need to eat; or simply leave on the plate what you don't need.

- **Leaving food on the plate is allowed even in your home.** Why should you eat in a day what you can eat in a week? Whether you have been invited for a meal, a party, a barbecue or you are having a relaxed Sunday lunch with wife and kids around the home, there is no need eat a lot of food.

- Your plate must not overflow with all cuts of meat and a variety of starches. Must one feel the tummy tight after every meal?

- Don't eat as if there is no food or a meal tomorrow or as if one has been starved for a week!

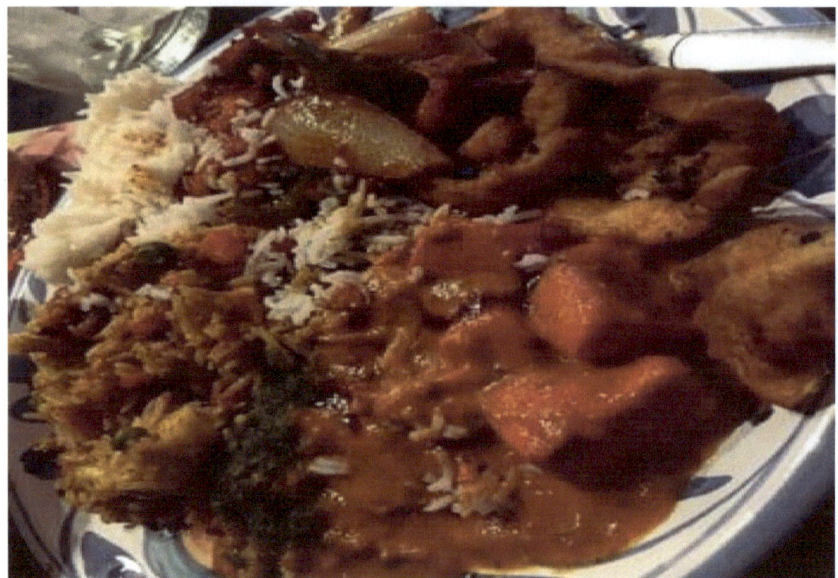

It is good to ask yourself questions when faced with food.

- Do I need an overflowing plate?

- Do I need that extra-large glass of wine?

- Why should I drink myself senseless?

The greed can be controlled. Make sensible choices of food at buffets and parties!

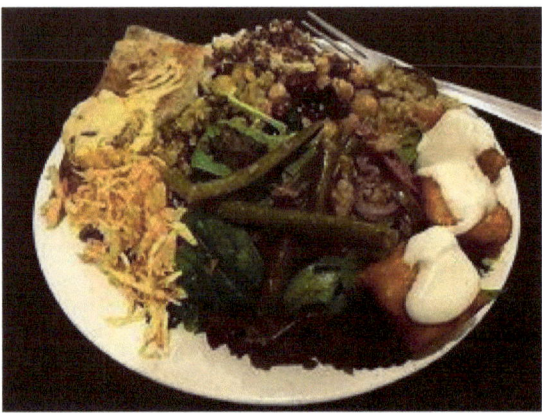

- Eat more greens. Vegetables do not make one fat, they add life!

- Eat lots of fruit.

Eat slowly and chew food thoroughly. That way one eats less.

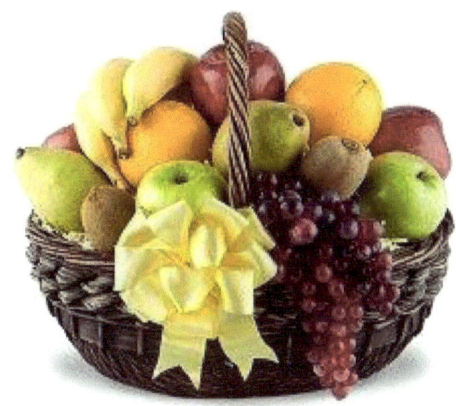

- Eat less of red meat and fatty meats as in beef and eat chicken and fish instead.
- Don't add extra salt to food. Salt slows movement of water in your body and encourages water to sit in your flesh. Don't drive when you can walk.
- Take walks around the block after work every day!
- Join the local gym and shed off the fat!

Enjoy good health! Don't carry unnecessary baggage!

Do not delay! Promote your own good health!

Engage in some Fitness exercise today! Learn to burn the food you take in by active work.Enjoy a healthy life! Exercise daily and lose unnecessary weight! invite a friend to work out with, take walks with or jog around the block. You could make it a routine with your spouse every day after work.
You sleep better after exercising!

YOU DON'T NEED A BAGFUL OF HEALTH PROBLEMS

Exercise!   Exercise!   Exercise!

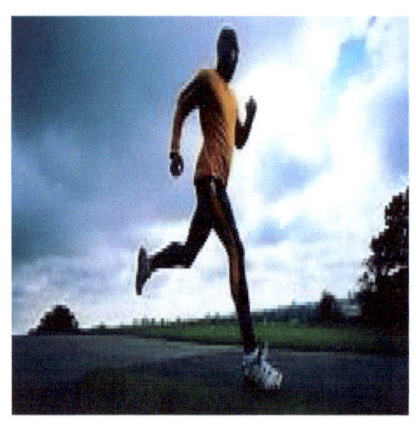

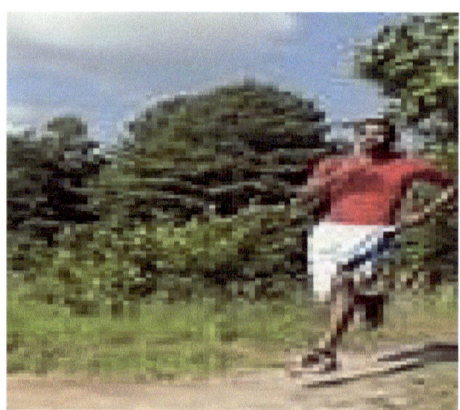

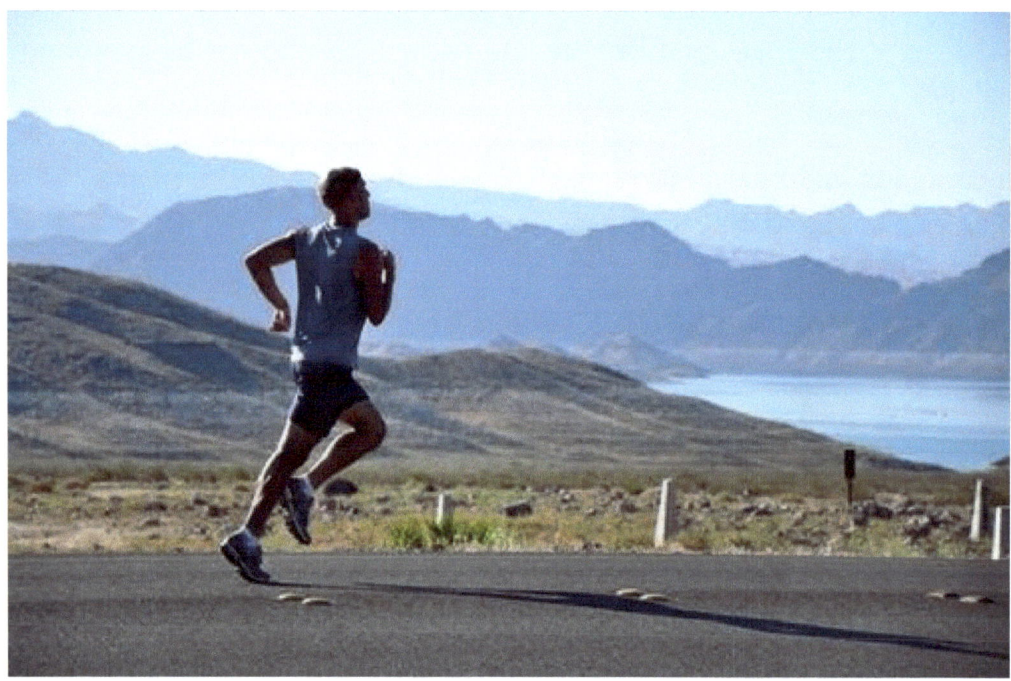

Exercise

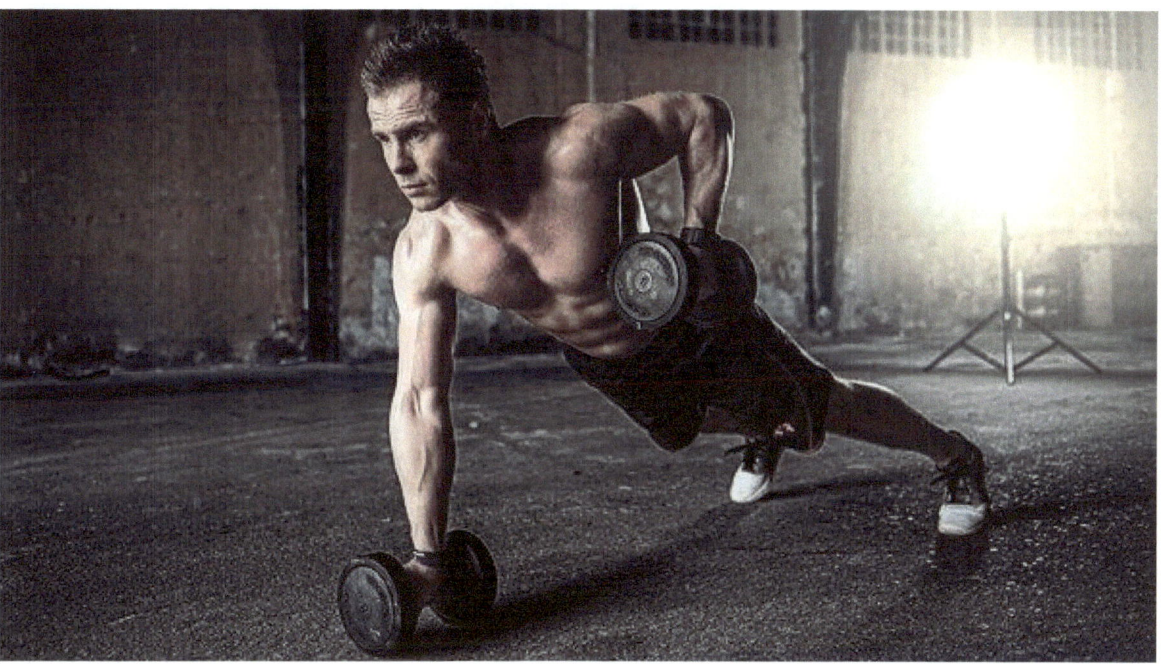

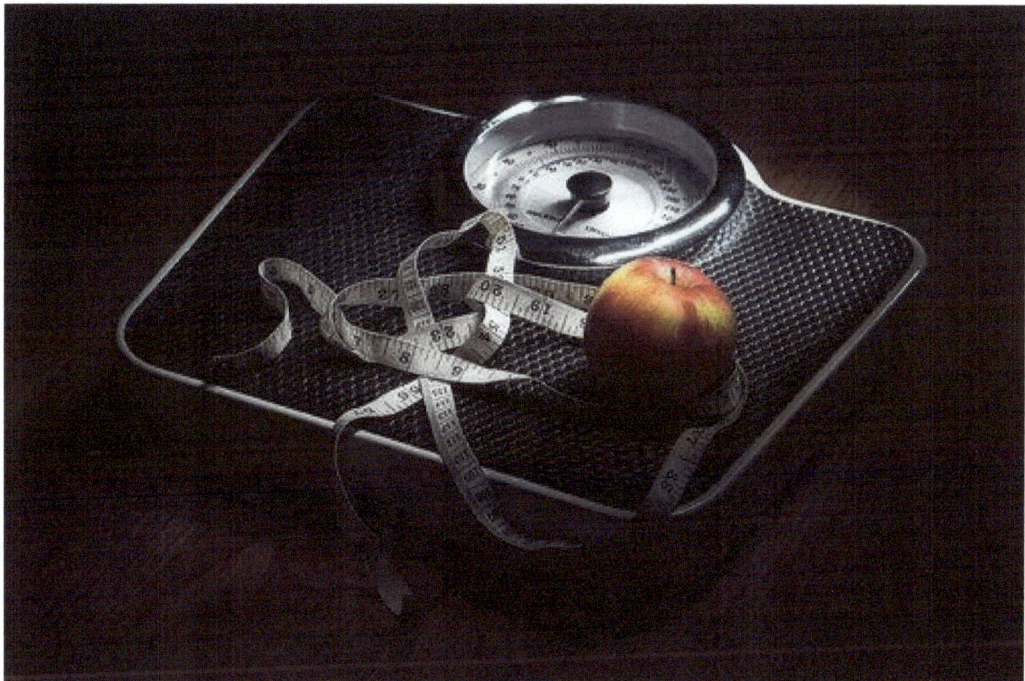

Lose the fat and flab and the unnecessary weight.

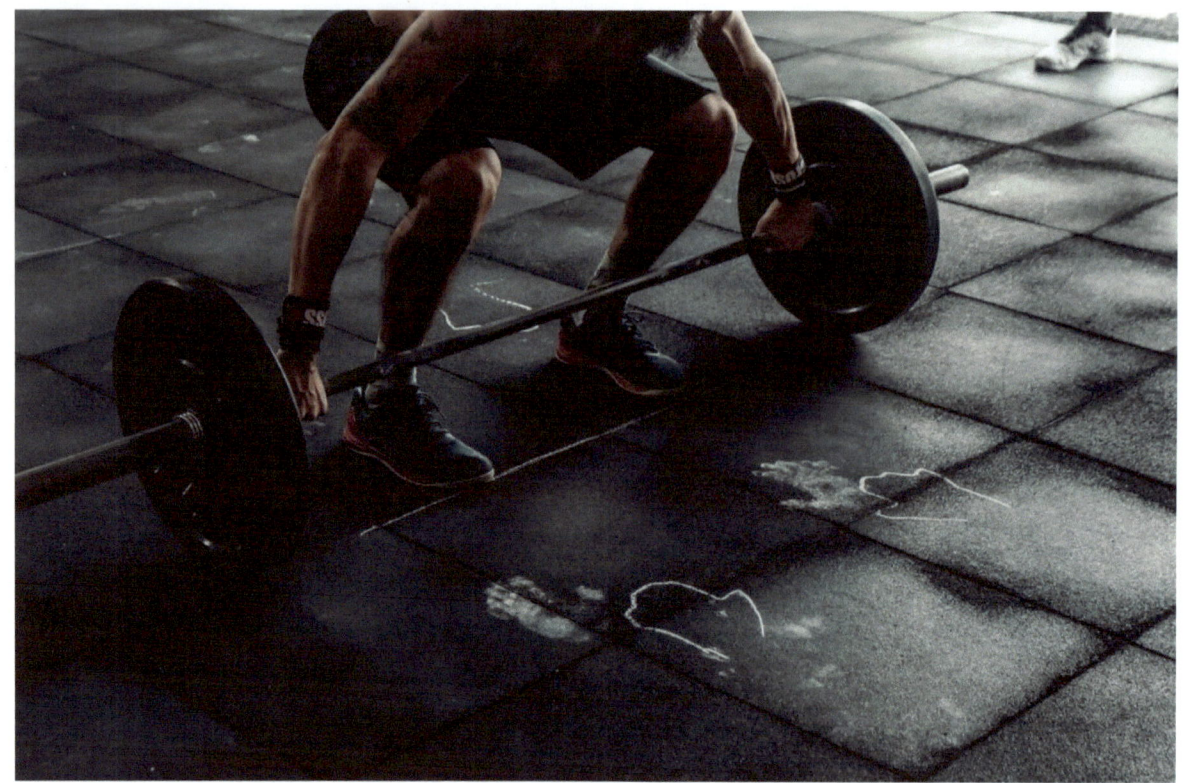

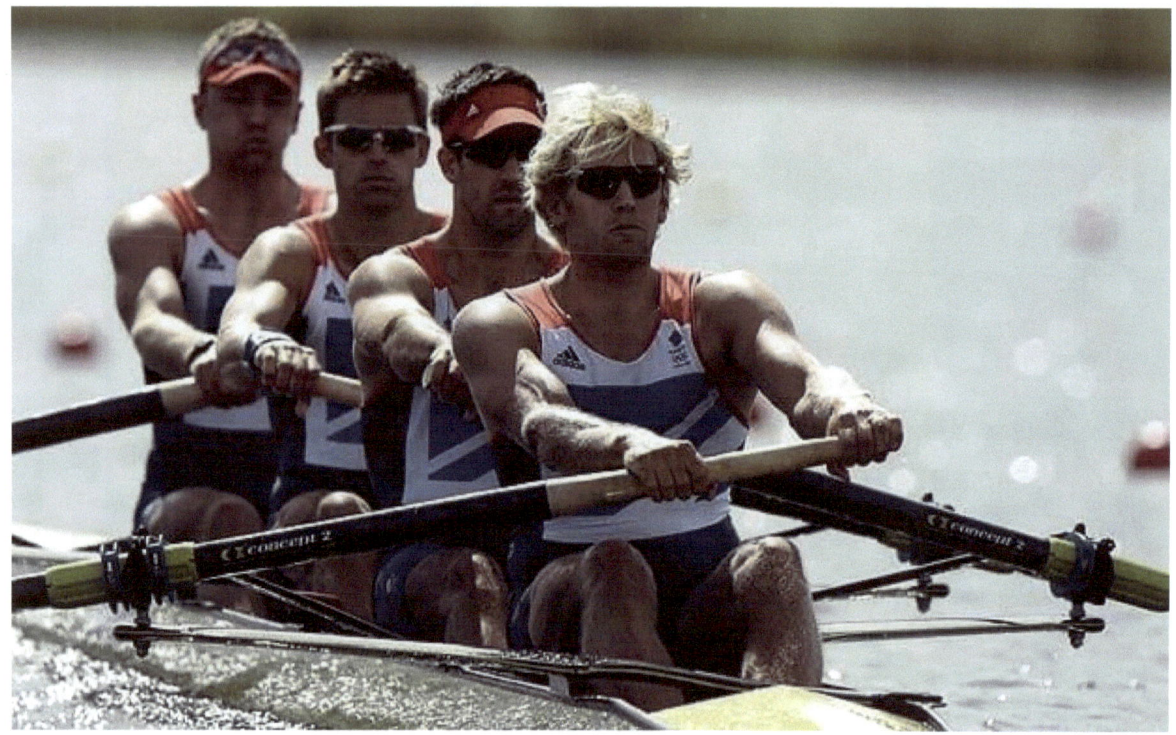

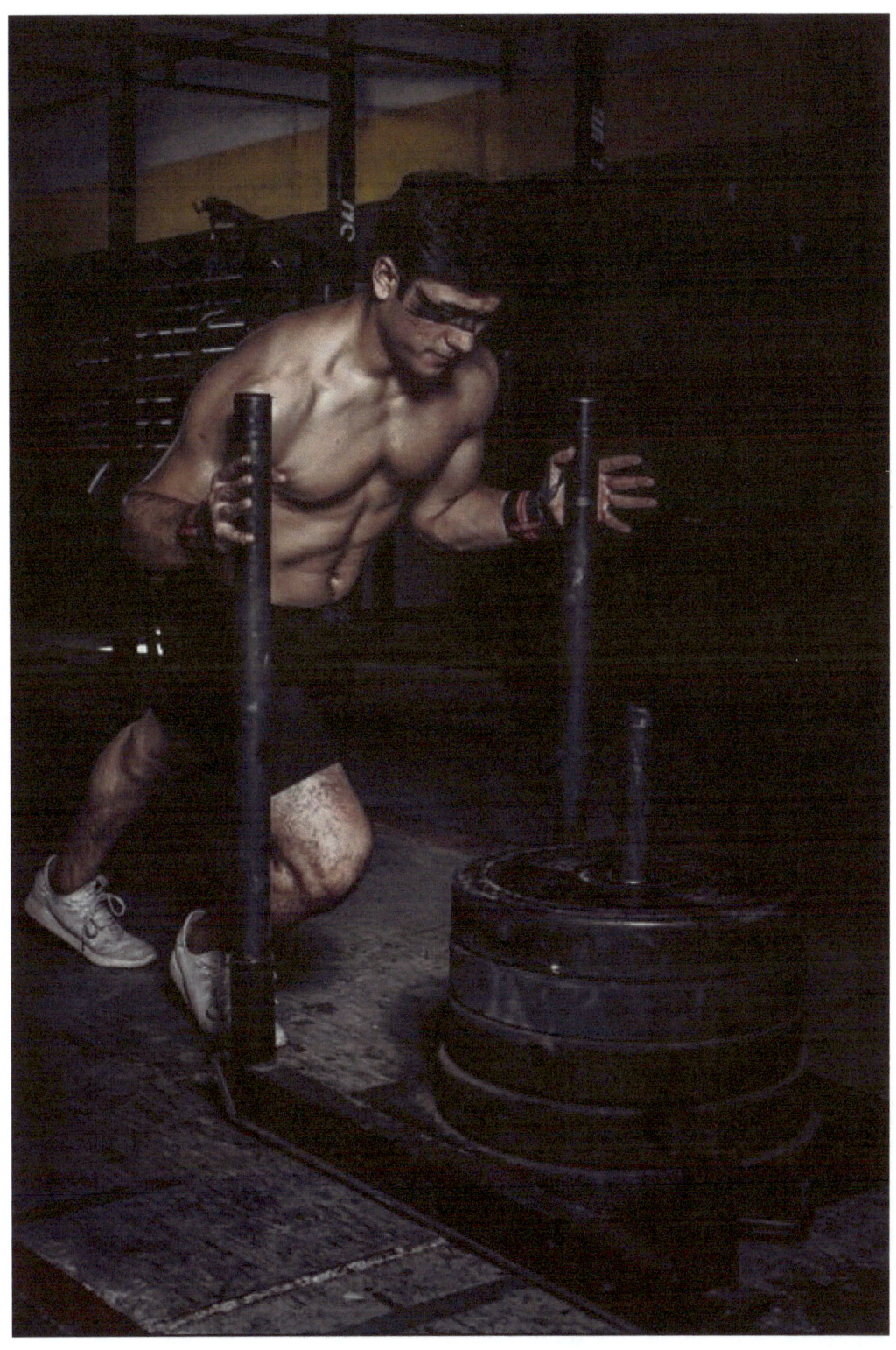

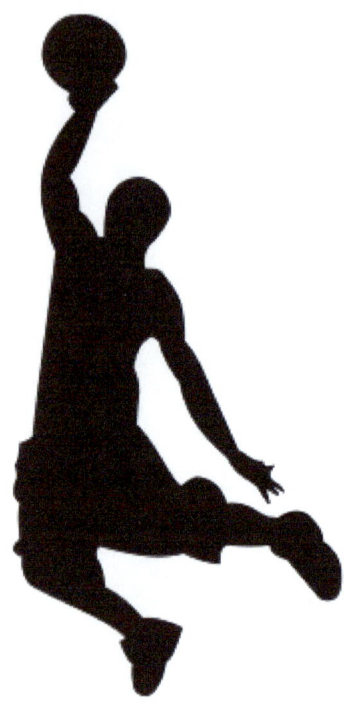

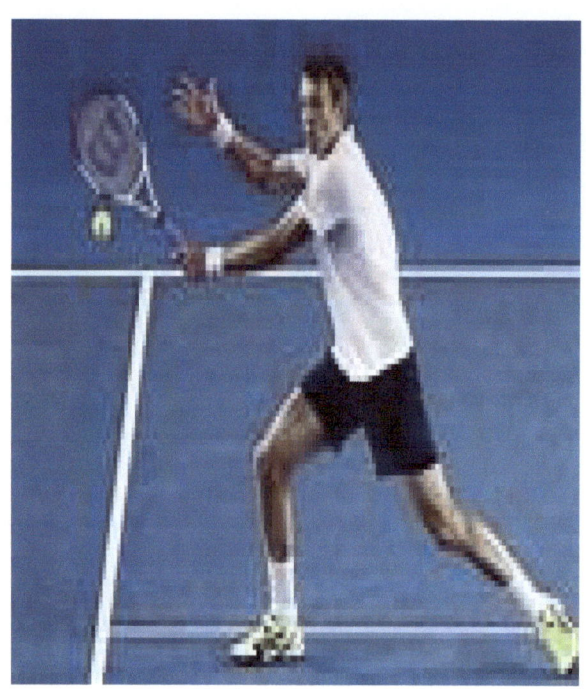

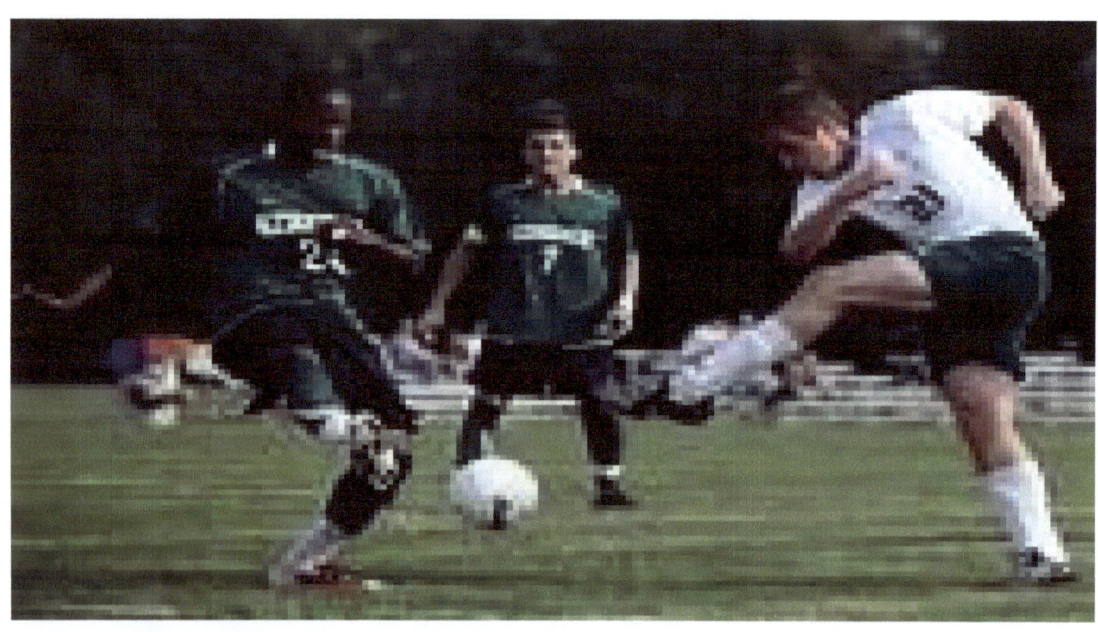

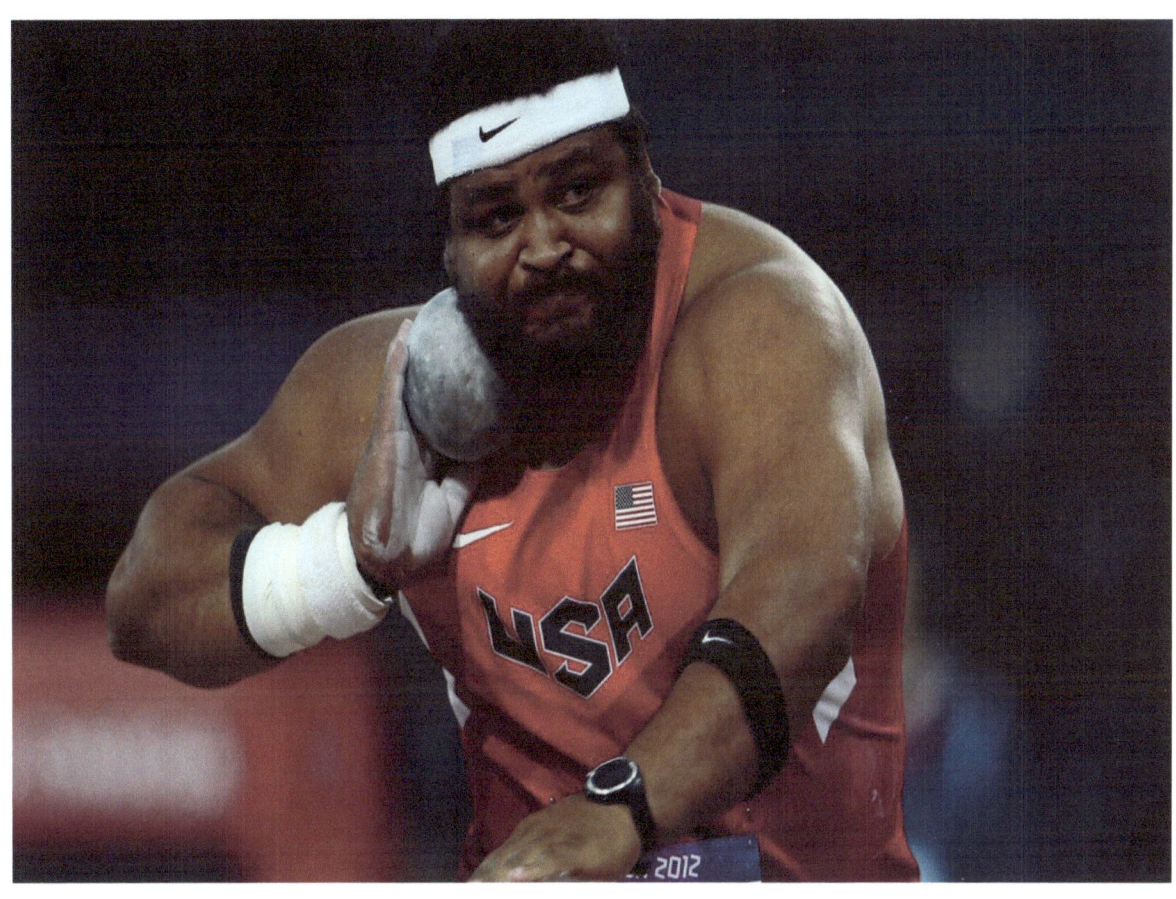

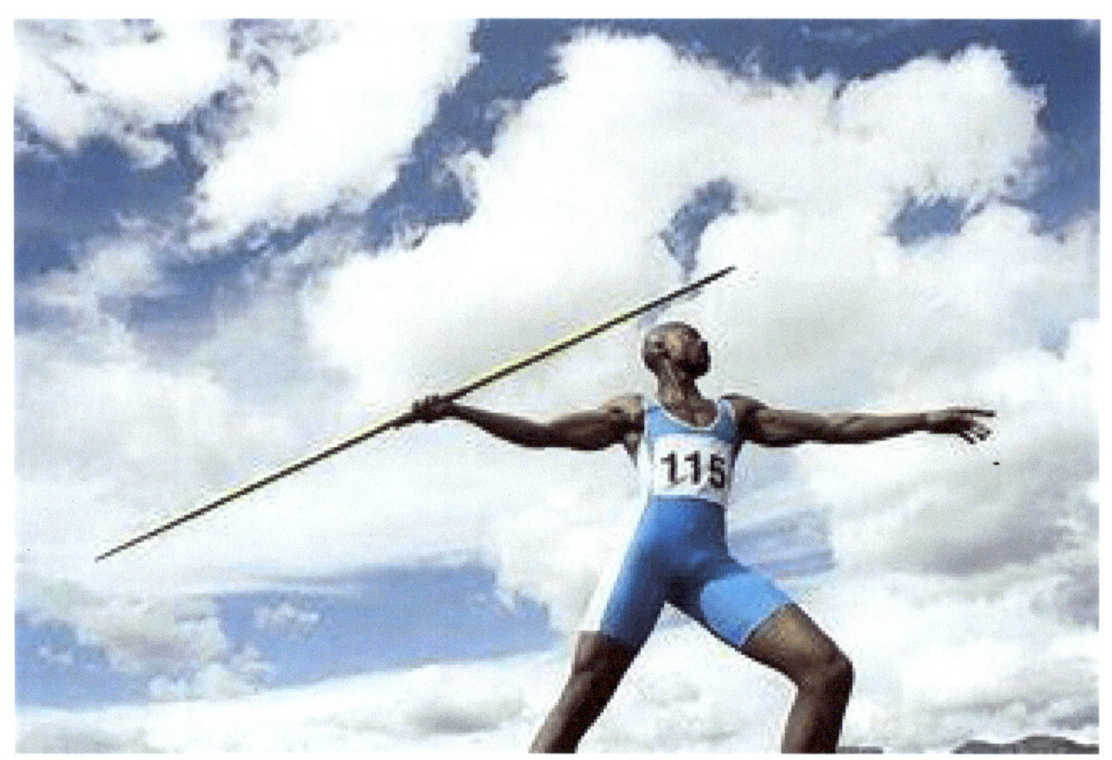

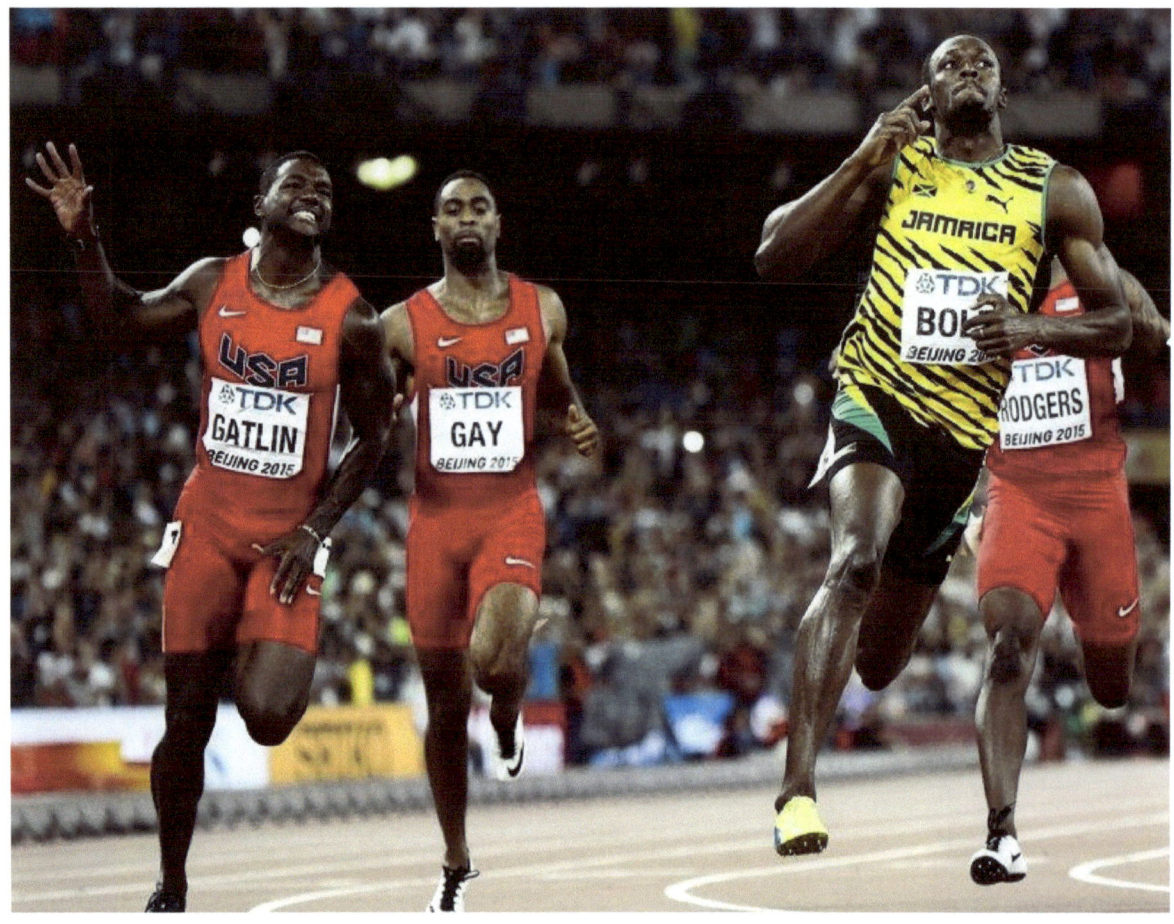

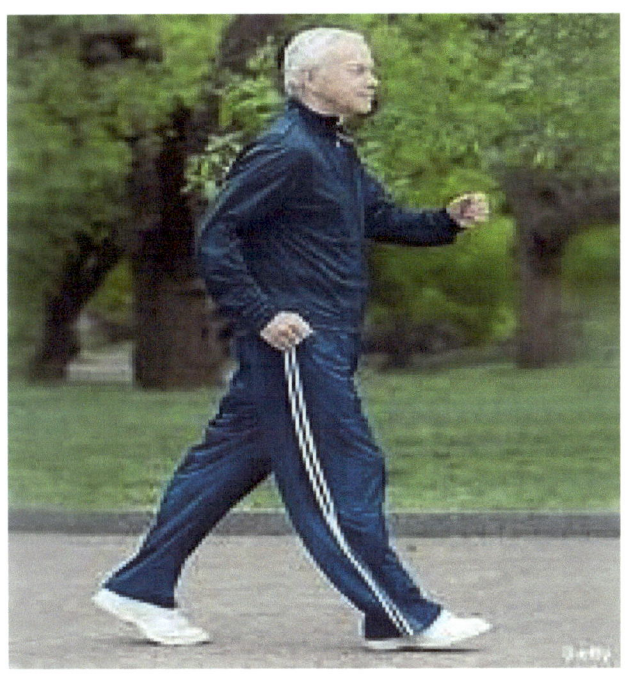

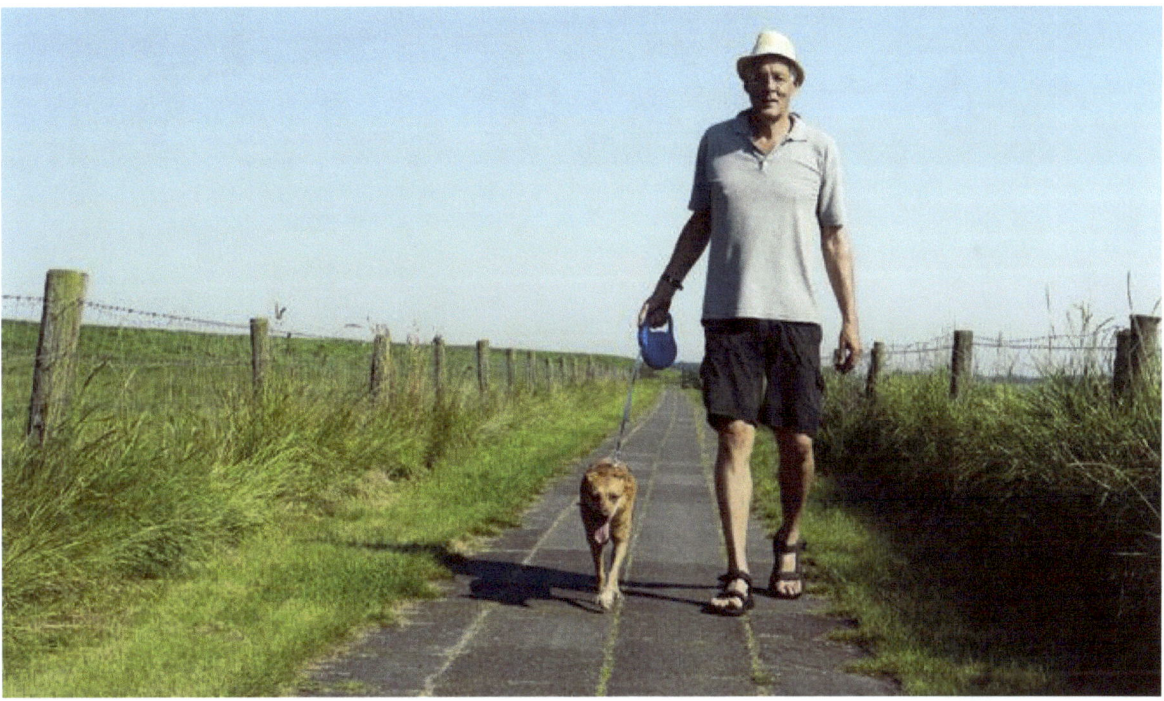

Walking everyday relieves stress, is healthy for your lungs, heart, body joints and muscle. Walking burns fat; makes your bowels move, and helps you sleep better!

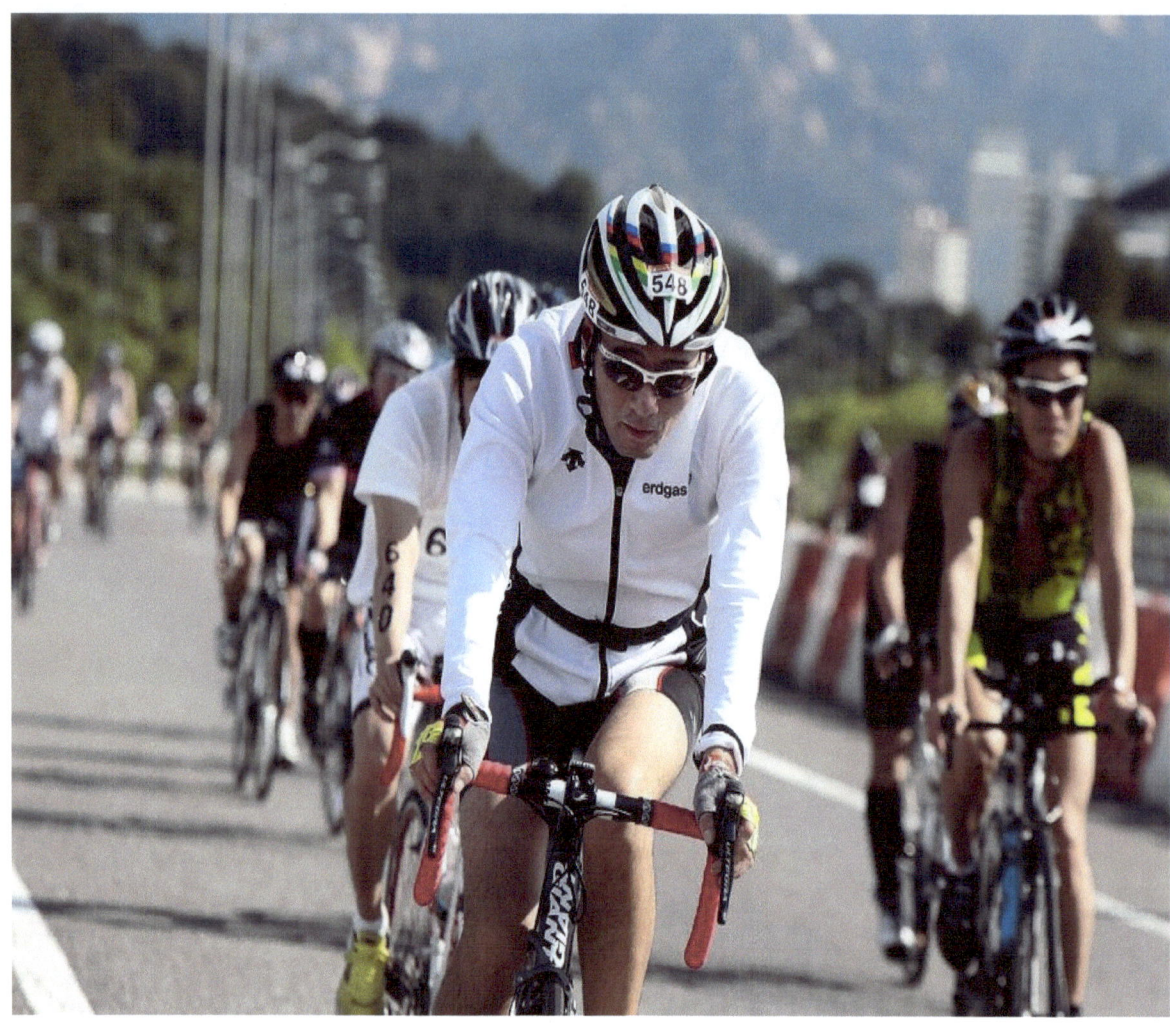

There is so much and a lot more to choose from to burn that unnecessary fat around your belly, your legs and give you a shapely healthy body!

MALE INFERTILITY

Infertility among men is least understood among many communities. For a long time, and in many cultures, male fertility has been taken for granted among men.

In some cultures, when a couple fails to achieve a pregnancy, the buck has almost always stopped with the woman. It is the woman who has been put under scrutiny and expected to undergo rituals to awaken her reproductive system. The man moves on and tries his luck with several women to prove his fertility. The impatience for fatherhood on the male side has resulted in extra-marital affairs, sexually transmitted infections, children out of wedlock who may or may not be revealed immediately, polygamous relationships and family disharmony. In many families, cases of infertility have ended up with marriage break up.

Men may associate infertility with poor sexual drive. Societal remedies for male infertility have centered on increasing sexual drive which takes many forms and activities thought to boost a man's virility.

A man's diet has always been a center of focus in boosting virility and may include additives thought to awaken his reproductive system, like high consumption of salt, cheese, and herbal mixtures. Please be aware that these substances and rituals do not stimulate or improve male fertility at all!

In some families the remedies have included an arrangement in which a brother fathers children on behalf of his brother, an arrangement that is kept a family secret. Women too have been known to source pregnancies from unknown sources when they suspect that the man is infertile. But it is not necessary for a couple to resort to these extremes before investigating their fertility status.

A couple is considered infertile after living together continuously for two years having regular normal sexual relationships at the right time of the female cycle.

Women are highly fertile for at least seven days from around the Fourteenth Day after a monthly period!

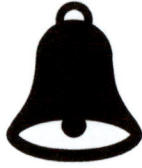

- The **female egg** is released from **the egg basket** or (ovary) around the fourteenth day after a period. This event is called (ovulation).

- **The egg is in the female's genital system** for at least seven days. This is the best time for a couple to try to achieve a pregnancy.

- The timing for the fertile days is very important as a couple may think that one of the partners could be infertile when the couple is trying for pregnancy at the wrong time of the month. Some couples withhold sexual activity for a day or two before this day to enhance their chances of a pregnancy.

- A woman can easily notice when she is fertile. The signs are:

    1. Her **vaginal secretions increase** and

    2. The secretions **become thinner and flowy.**

    3. The woman's **body temperature rises towards ovulation.**

It means it is necessary for a woman to check her temperature every morning before brushing her teeth or having an early cup of coffee. The couple must get a

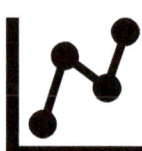

thermometer and learn how to read body temperature.

- The problem of failing to achieve a pregnancy can occur where partners live separately and meet once a month or where one partner has a job that takes him or her away for a while.

What is male fertility?

Male fertility is determined by ability to produce normal and adequate numbers of male seed (spermatozoa).

- It is estimated that normal sperm count should be over 50 million sperms per millilitre of semen. Figures below this count may result in male sterility.

- The male seed must have a normal size, a normal shape and must be able to swim to meet the female egg and fertilize it.

- Only one sperm (male seed) fertilizes the egg but sperm are required in large numbers to produce a substance that makes the egg soft to enable one sperm to fertilize the egg.

What may cause one to produce a small amount of sperms or no sperms at all?

1.Inadequate hormones.

- Men may have problems in producing adequate amounts of testicular stimulating hormone which stimulates testicular cells to produce the male hormone testosterone. This hormone testosterone is essential in the production of the male seed and maturation of the male seed.

- The male tubes male be blocked by previous infection and the male seed fails to reach the woman.

- The testes need adequate amounts of Follicle Stimulating Hormone from the lower part of the brain (Pituitary gland) to produce sperms.

- Inadequate stimulation of the testes by the hormone results in low production of sperms. The second hormone from the pituitary gland (ICSH) Interstitial Cell Stimulating Hormone) causes production of the male hormone testosterone by the testes.

- Testosterone causes the male seed to mature. In the absence of adequate amounts of testosterone, sperms are fragile and may not have a normal shape, size and ability to swim vigorously.

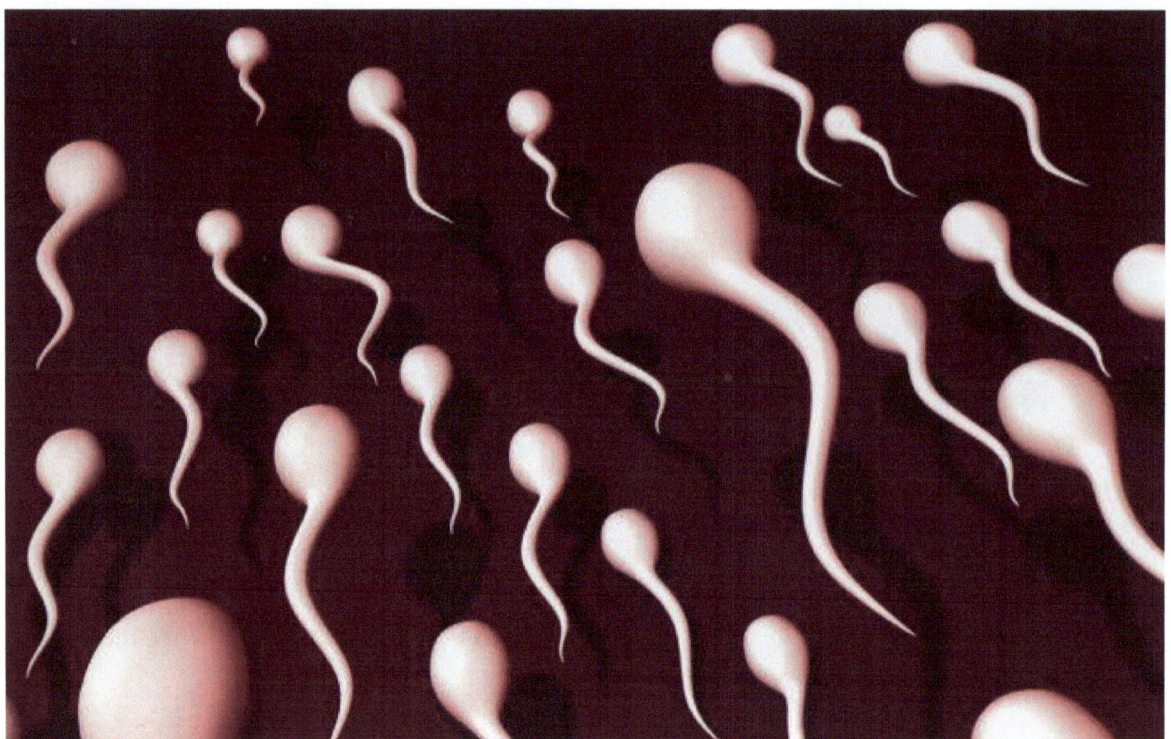

2.Blockage in the testes

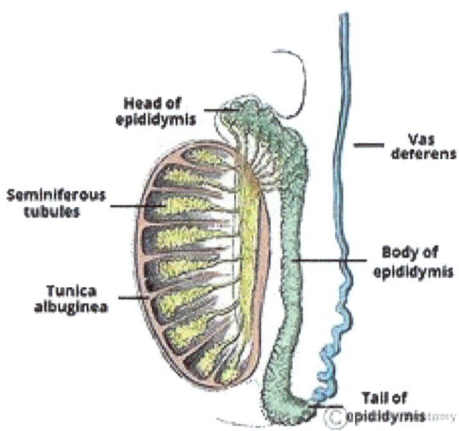

Sexually transmitted infections may leave testes swollen or the tubes that ferry the male seed blocked by pus and when healing occurs, the tissues stick together, form scars and block the flow of sperms making the individual sterile or infertile.

- It is important that one avoids sexually transmitted diseases through having one faithful sexual partner or using a condom. In the event of one partner getting sexually transmitted disease,
- Both partners must be treated thoroughly until the course of antibiotics is finished and must be tested to prove they have been treated and are free from the infection.

How can a man tell that he is infertile?

- Using one's eyes to examine the colour or thickness of one's semen **will not tell** that one is fertile or not.
- One's organs are examined to see if they are normal and they are not blocked.
- Investigations on the flow of hormones, (hormonal assays), are done. Specimens of blood are collected to check the amounts of the male hormone **(testosterone)** one's body is producing. Low levels of the male hormone may mean that the male organs may fail to produce adequate numbers of the male seed.
- Specimens of one's semen are examined by powerful machines in laboratories.
- A sperm count is done to assess the amount of the male seed. A man must produce millions of sperms in a drop of semen. Low numbers of sperm counts may reduce the chances of a pregnancy being achieved. Few sperms limit the chances of fertilization of the female egg.
- The shape of the male seed is examined. Deformed sperms maybe unable to fertilize the female egg. Deformed sperms are usually weak and fail to reach the female egg to fertilize it.
- The ability and strength to swim fast enough to fertilize the female egg. Sluggish or lazy sperms may not swim fast enough to fertilize an egg.

It is important to understand that discharging large amounts of semen does not mean that a man is fertile. It is the amount of seed and the quality of seed in that fluid that determines fertility.

- Semen is a fluid that transports the male seed.
- Semen may not contain the male seed if the testes fail to produce the seed. The amount of water in a river does not determine the number of fish in it!
- Some semen is produced by testicular tissue and most of it is produced by the prostate gland.

What can one do?

Relaxation, relaxation, relaxation! Tension, extreme anxiety, are bad for making babies! Let your body and mind be at ease. Don't talk about your wishes! Get the thoughts of having a baby right at the back of your mind and don't bring them forward while love-making. Let the body do its natural processes in a relaxed manner. Couples thought to be infertile have been surprised to find they have a baby on the way years after trying for a baby.

Get your mind occupied find a hobby, something that changes your focus.

- It cannot be over-emphasized that a couple must live together continuously while trying for a pregnancy.
- Have access to information on the female cycle and time the sexual activity at the times of the month when the female partner is most fertile.
- Several investigations of both male and female reproductive systems are done to exclude infections, blockages and tumours of the genital organs.
- Supplementary hormones can be given to any of the partners who may not be producing adequate amounts of hormones. Low hormonal flow can be stimulated by supplements prescribed by health specialists.
- The female system is examined. It is important to ascertain if the flow of the female hormones is adequate to enable the ovaries to produce the female egg.

- Assisted fertility can be discussed between the couple and an obstetrician to enable a couple to achieve a pregnancy.

After these tests, is it possible to be a father?

- Blockage of any part of the testes cannot be reversed. There are alternatives available to becoming a father through artificial methods after the above tests identify the cause of infertility.
- Details of artificial methods of achieving fatherhood can be discussed with the health specialists after they have investigated on possible causes of infertility.

.

SMOKING AND YOUR HEALTH

SO, YOU SMOKE?

Smoking is a **<u>habit learnt and nurtured by an individual</u>** for reasons best known to the individual. Adolescents may try smoking in a bid to be noticed, to win friends, to appear cool and different and out of curiosity.

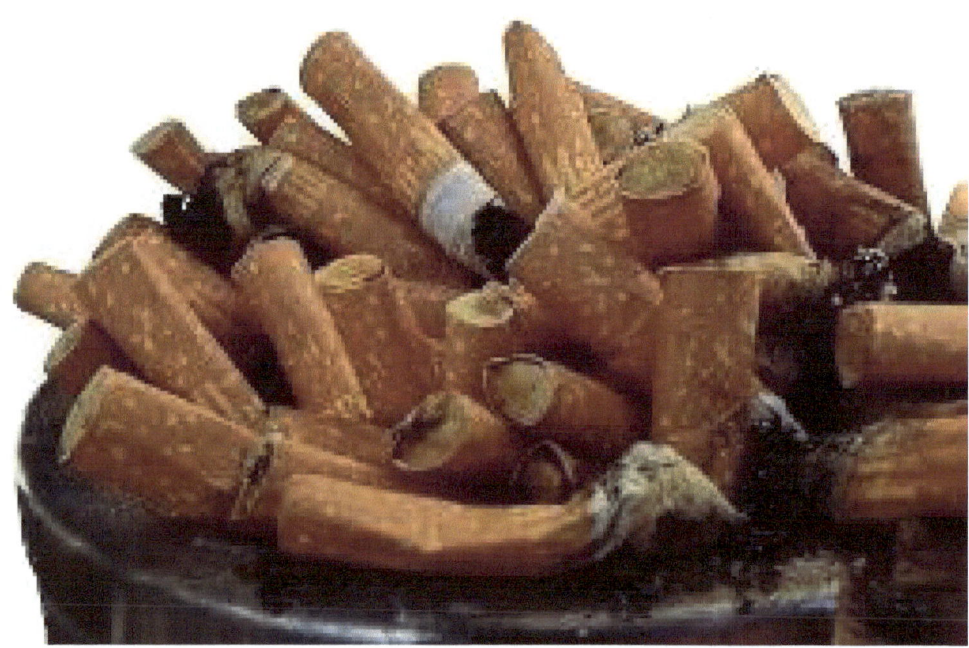

Excuses for smoking

Adult smokers come up with many lame excuses for perpetuating their bad habit of smoking.

A smoker may call his bad habit 'socializing', but smoking is at the expense of one's health.

A smoker may call the habit a means to reduce boredom.

Young people may feel it is being cool and with it to smoke.

Some young people may have grown up around smokers and are inducted into smoking.

Lack of good role models may result in a young person trying bad habits.

Feeling of belonging and avoiding being the odd one out.

Smokers may come up with as many reasons as they can, but the truth is there is absolutely nothing to gained by smoking instead, the smoker is slowly destroying his lungs and shortening his life!

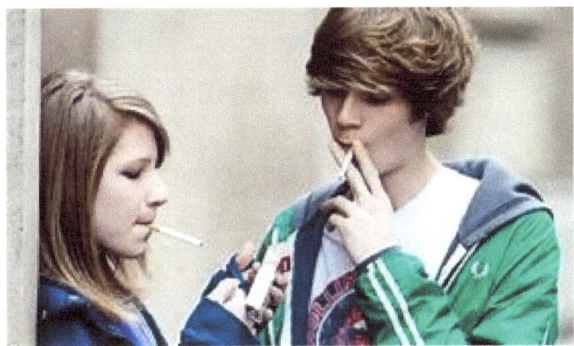

Some smokers think that smoking helps in reduction of nervousness and bolsters courage to speak and strength to work.

All these excuses are false. That is called **addiction**.

Cigarettes contain a substance or poison called **nicotine**; a smoker's body will crave for more nicotine once one is hooked to smoking. Nicotine is habit forming.

A smoker must smoke to keep the levels of nicotine in the body high and craves for more and slowly one cannot do without it. Nicotine gives a hangover or craving for more smoking.

Smokers think puffing away a cigarette heats up the body on a cold day. This too is false. None of the above excuses are true.

Facts about smoking

Smoking is habit forming. Once one starts smoking, there is a tendency to continue smoking because the body craves for more and more nicotine.

Smoking gives one a false feeling of satisfaction and yet it imprisons a person and ties the person down to smoking.

Smoke is absorbed into the body tissues so that one's body and all body fluids like saliva, urine, sweat, smell of cigarettes.
One's breath smells of smoke.

Smoking sinks into teeth and changes their color permanently.

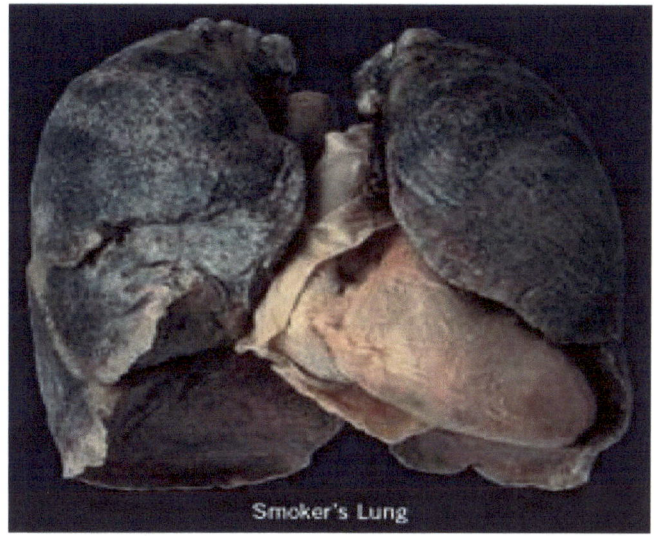
Smoker's Lung

Smoking and health

- Smoke goes to the lungs where it forms an oily sticky tarry paste on lung tissue weakening the lung tissue and reducing the lungs' ability to absorb fresh air. That is the beginning of lung diseases and breathing problems that are likely to end one's life!

- **Smoking reduces absorption of air by lung tissue thus reducing oxygen circulation** in the body.

- Smoke weakens lung tissue and causes a lingering, wet, loud cough, **chronic bronchitis**.

- A smoker has increased chances of suffering from lung infections such as pneumonias, tuberculosis, cancer of the lungs and lung collapse.

- Cigarette smoke can cause ***asthmatic attack*** and ***heart attack*** in bystanders or members of the family.

- Smoking causes narrowing and hardening of blood vessels causing ***high blood pressure***. Narrowing of blood vessels that supply the heart slows down supply of blood to the heart tissue increasing the chances of ***heart failure.***

Smoking and your social status

- A smoker's clothes smell of cigarettes even after washing them. The smell can be extremely unpleasant in the presence of non-smokers.

- **Cigarette smoke coats one's teeth and they are stained into varied shades of grey** that no toothpaste can completely remove.

- The lips, tongue and mouth are coated grey.

- A smoker's breath has strong cigarette smell making close ups and whispers very unpleasant even after using smokers' toothpaste!

- Smoking has the risk of fires. A cigarette stub left burning can destroy everything one has worked for all his life, other people's properties, vegetation and even innocent lives!

Passive smoking

Smokers tend to be insensitive of others' preferences.

Puffing away cigarette smoke, in a crowded place, in the presence of babies and children, wife, friends, fellow passengers in a bus, in a plane or room, forces everyone within reach to inhale the smoke. This is forcing everyone within the reach of the smoke to be a passive smoker.

Passive smoking is more dangerous than active smoking because active smokers exhale the smoke while passive smokers keep the smoke deep in their lungs.

It is extremely selfish to make other people uncomfortable through one's bad habits. If a smoker cares about other people, his family included, then he must do everybody a favor and smoke outside the house and away from the general public.

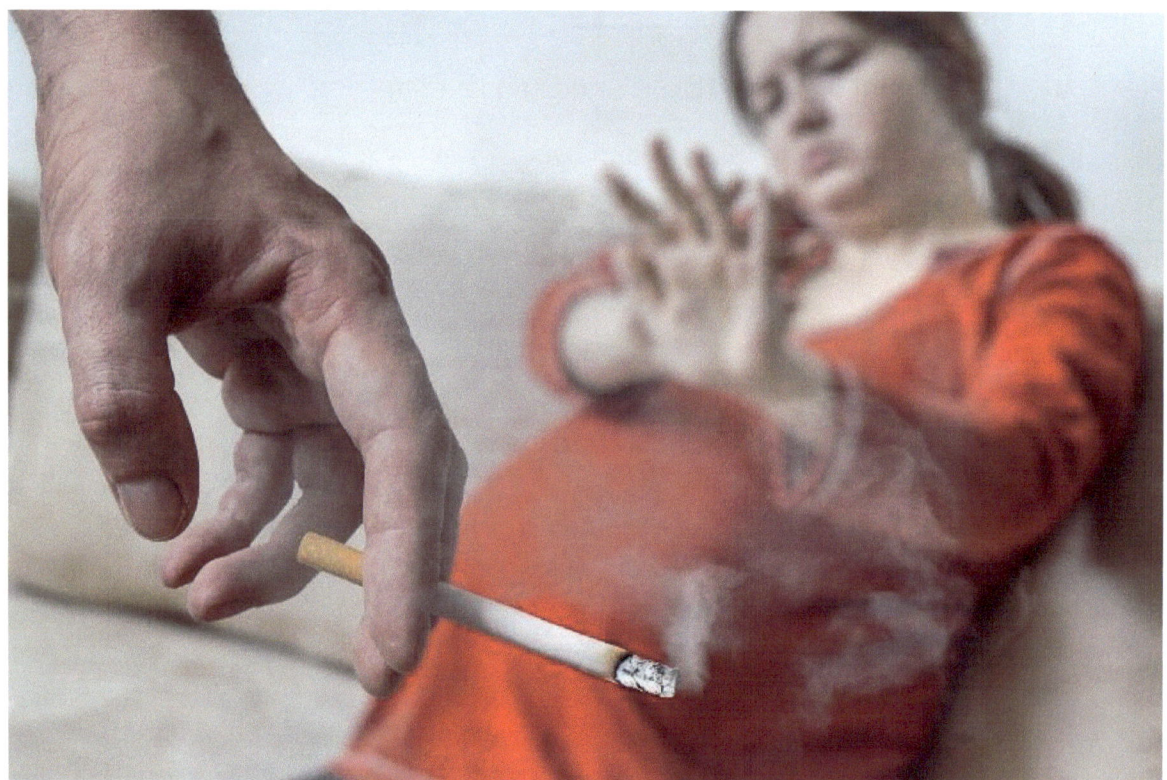

SMOKING AND PREGNANCY

Smoking narrows blood vessels and therefore reduces blood flow to the placenta, a structure attached to the mother's blood system and connected to the baby by the umbilical cord, which provides food and air to the unborn baby and protects the baby from infections.

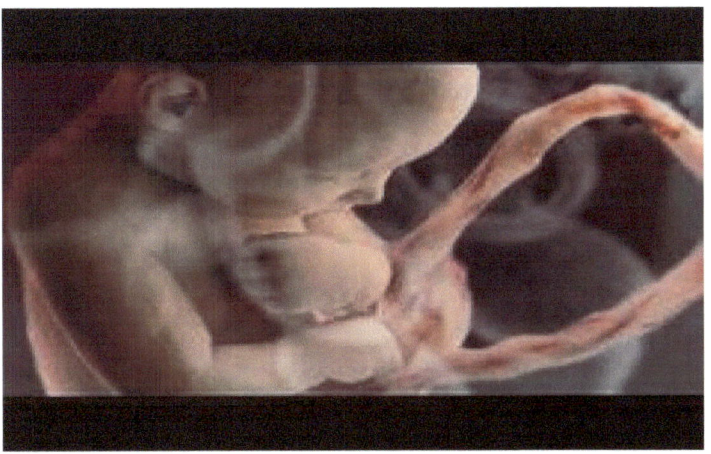

Reduced blood flow to the placenta reduces oxygen and nutrients to the unborn child slowing down the growth of the unborn child. A smoking pregnant mother can easily go into premature labor. There are increased chances of ectopic pregnancy miscarriages, kidney damage to the baby, sudden infant death and birth defects. The baby may also have ear, nose and throat problems. The baby is born small for dates. The baby is likely to develop breathing problems at birth, and almost always will need resuscitation at birth.

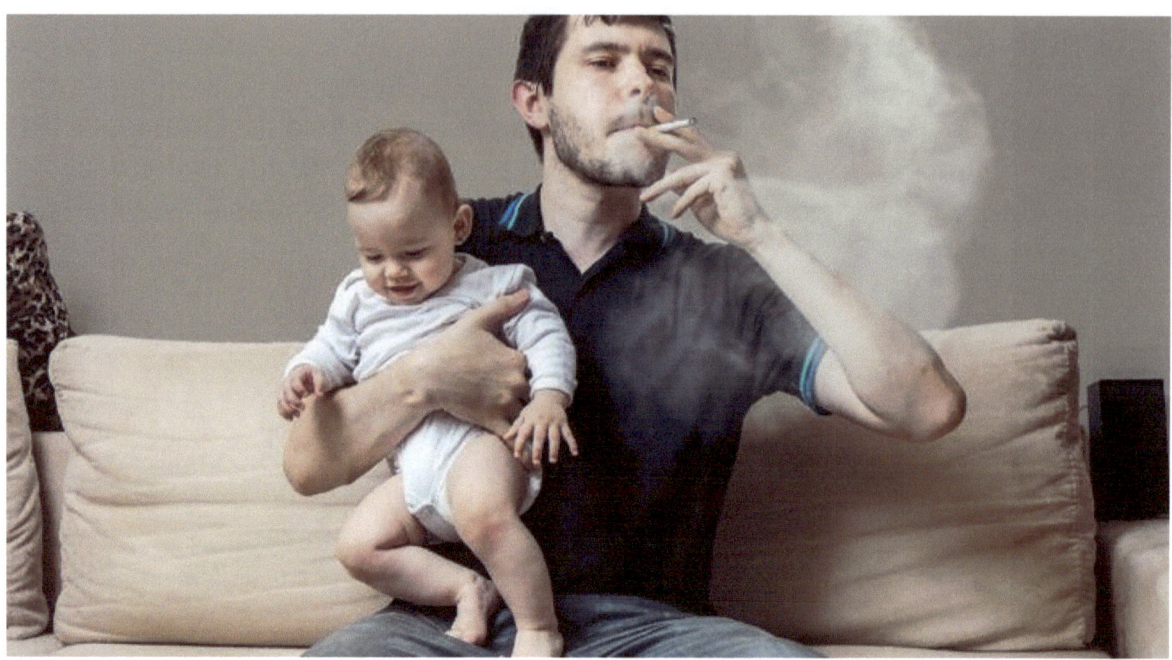

Why are you smoking the baby?

A baby exposed to smoke everyday may develop upper respiratory diseases. The baby may be lost due to difficulty in breathing.

The baby is in danger of cigarette burns.

If you smoke as a couple, it is time you thought about the harm you are causing to your unborn child and the rest of the family!

Reasons for quitting smoking

Smoking kills! That is a true proven fact. By continuing to smoke, you shorten your life by many years.

Smoking is expensive. There are better things to do with your that will not you're your health. From today, get a piggy bank and for every packet of cigarettes you buy, drop an equal amount of money in the piggy bank. Open the piggy bank at the end of a month or whenever you choose and see how much money you have burnt to destroy your lungs.

If you saved all the money you spend on cigarettes per month you could buy many loaves of bread for the needy like orphans, you could engage in a small income generating project with the money!

There is nothing to gain from smoking; one merely burns money and burns life away!

What can one do to gradually reduce the craving for smoking?

The decision to stop smoking is entirely yours! Once you make up your mind that you want to stop smoking:

- Throw away everything that reminds you of a cigarette such as a cigarette lighter, ashtray and clear your garden or apartment of cigarette stubs.

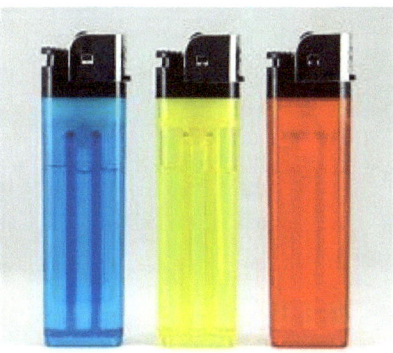

- Don't buy cigarettes.

- Don't ask anybody, stranger of friend for a cigarette.

- Don't accept an offer of a cigarette. Tell all your friends you have stopped smoking.

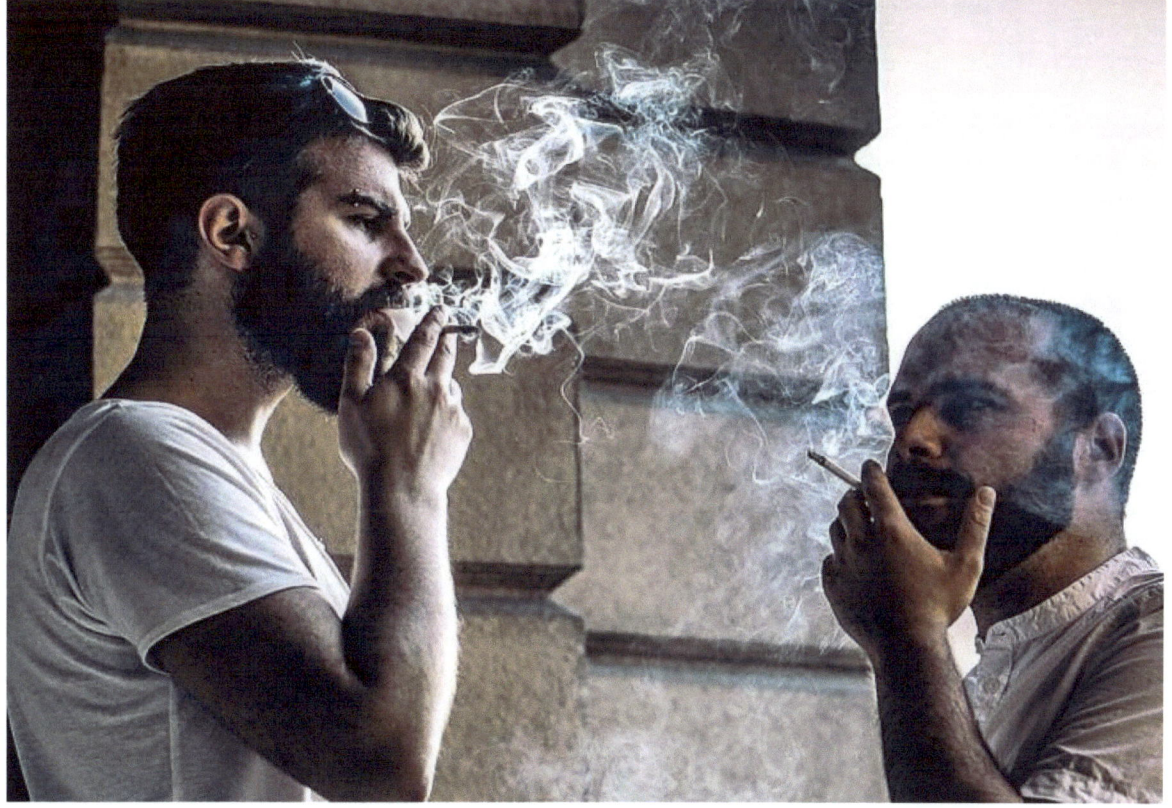

- Thwart the craving for a cigarette with an apple, a sweet or snacks, peanuts or better still some small chore or exercise.

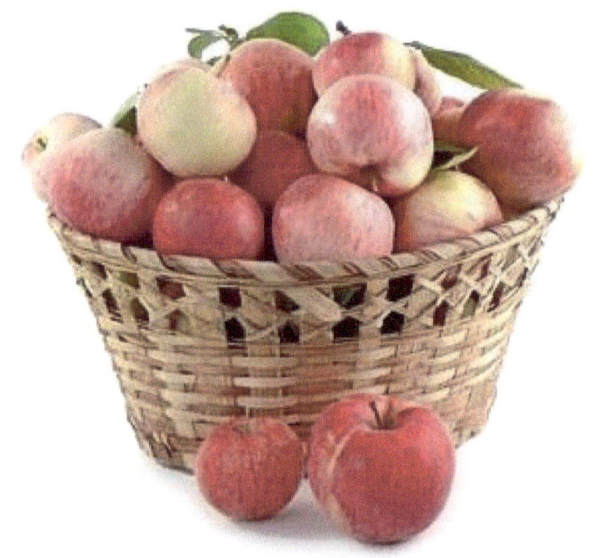

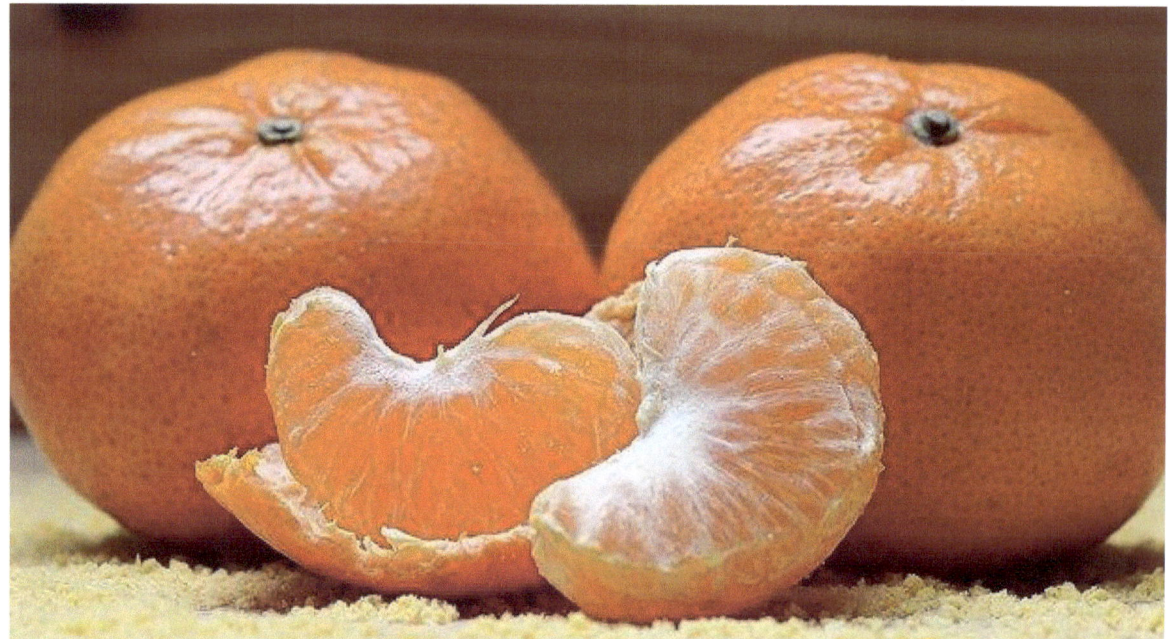

- You can purchase smoke cessation patches from your pharmacy

Engage yourself in other hobbies, pastimes that lift your spirits up, something that you can measure your achievement and success at the end of the day.

How about an income generating project? Surely you need extra cash!

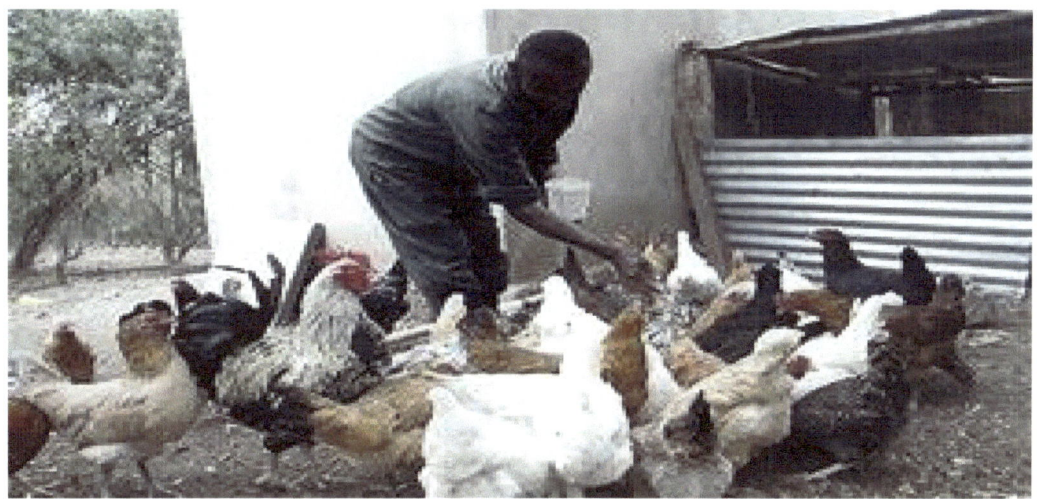

Get your hands busy with something productive.

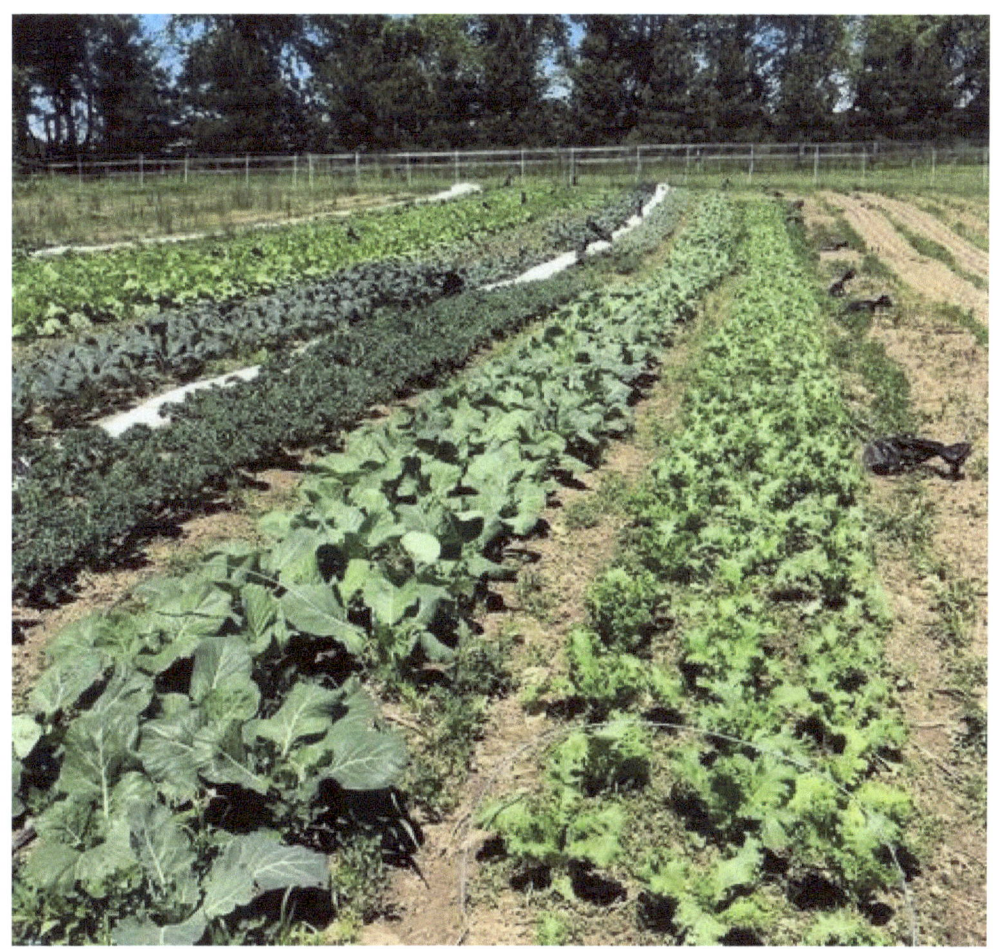

- Help an elderly person do his garden, clean her house.
- Get involved in charity work, join the Red Cross.
- Engage in a sport.
  Travel and see the world instead of burning the money and destroying your health.
- Keep young people occupied and out of trouble by engaging them in sport, holding art classes etc.

Cigarette stubs left smoldering have caused some of the devastating fires, destroying houses, nurture and obliterating whole neighborhoods?

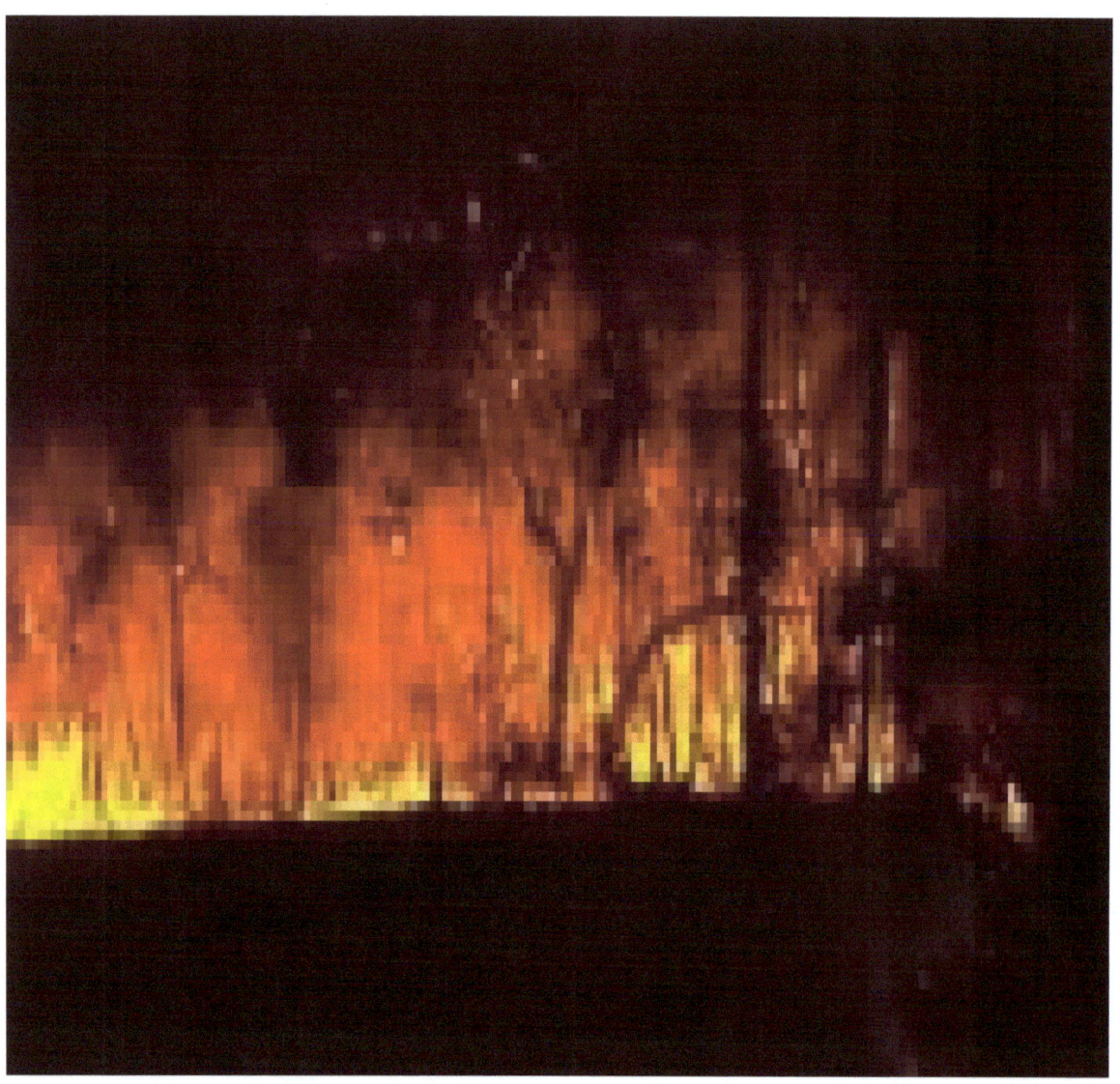

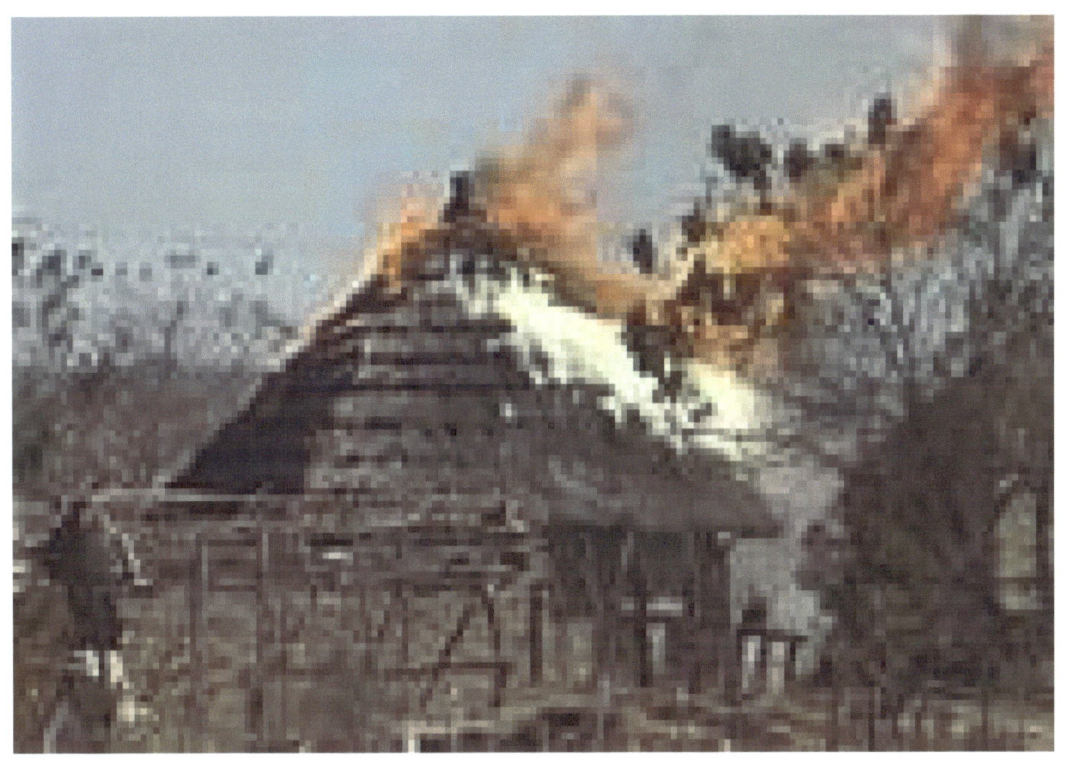

STOP SMOKING AND LIVE LONGER TO ENJOY YOUR LIFE!

CONTRIBUTE TO A CLEAN AND SAFE ENVIROMENT FREE OF CIGERRETE STUBS AND SMOKE!

YOUR QUESTIONS ANSWERED

Ask **BABA** any questions about your health and you will get the responses in the next issue!

If you have comments to make about any topic discussed in this magazine, drop a line to BABA Men's health magazine.

Write to the editor, E-mail:babamagazine@gmail.com

The Editor,

Q. How can I prove that my sperms are strong and that I am fertile?

A. A healthy young person who has had healthy secondary sexual development and has not experienced infections of the genital system should not have undue fears about fertility neither should he need to prove anything about fertility to anyone. These anxieties should not put pressure on young people to find an excuse for indulging in unplanned, illicit and wanton sexual behaviors. Proof of fertility will be seen when one is ready to start a family. Should one have a problem then, health personnel will conduct the necessary investigations and provide relevant advice and remedy where possible.

Q. Is the appearance of one's semen suggestive of one's fertility status?

A. The semen is fluid which provides a medium and transport for the male seed from the testicles through the male reproductive system. The male seed cannot be seen with the naked eye. Sperms can only be seen under a microscope. Looking at the semen cannot provide anyone with answers about fertility. Tests on fertility are done in adults after a doctor's advice and consent.

Q. What if one produces small amounts of semen; is this cause for concern?

A. One may produce any amount of semen but what is important is the health of the actual seed contained in the semen which can only be seen in laboratories by specialists using special equipment.

Editor's Profile

Dr. Nester Kadzviti Murira was born in Mhondoro, in Zimbabwe. She went to Zowa Mupatsi, and Tendai Government School for Primary Education. She attended the Salvation Army Usher Secondary School in Zimbabwe.

Nester graduated with a PhD in Health from Birmingham City University UK, a Masters' Degree in Medical Education from the University of Dundee, Scotland, a Diploma in Nurse Education and a Bachelors' Degree in Adult Education from the University of Zimbabwe. She received research training at Stockholm, Uppsala and Umea Universities in Sweden, and University of Sheffield, England. She is an RN and a Midwife.

Nester taught at Women's University in Africa and in the Ministry of Health Nurse Training Schools in Zimbabwe. She worked as a Research Midwife at the University of Zimbabwe and in rural District Hospitals, in Provincial and Tertiary hospitals in Zimbabwe. In Private Practice she opened one of the first Nurse managed HIV/AIDS Nursing Homes in Zimbabwe, Midwifery-run Maternity Home and established a Domiciliary Midwifery Service in Harare, Zimbabwe.

Nester is a founder member of the Africa Midwives Research Network AMRN, now LAMRN. She is a published researcher, an author of several Health Education books for all ages, textbooks for health professionals, children's books and is also a film script writer and copywriter.

She is the Editor of FEMALEA magazine and Maternal Morbidity and Mortality Journal for Sub-Saharan African Midwives.

NEXT MONTH

Hernias

Why do I have one sex of children?

Sexually Transmitted Infections